WIRED FOR SOUND

A JOURNEY INTO HEARING

Beverly Biderman

Trifolium Books Inc.

Toronto, Canada

Trifolium Books Inc.
250 Merton Street, Suite 203
Toronto, Ontario, Canada M4S 1B1

Trifolium Books Inc. acknowledges with graditude the generous support of the
Government of Canada's Publishing Industry Development Program (BPIDP).

Canadian Cataloguing in Publication Data
Biderman, Beverly, 1946–
         Wired for sound : a journey into hearing

Includes bibliographical references and index.
ISBN 1-895579-32-5

1. Biderman, Beverly, 1946– . 2. Cochlear implants.
3. Deaf — Canada — Biography
I. Title.

RF305.B52 1998   617.8'9   C98-930269-5

Printed and bound in Canada
10 9 8 7 6 5 4 3 2 1

Editor: Wendy Thomas
Design: Heidy Lawrance Associates
Project coordinator: Rodney Burke

Ordering Information
*Orders by Canadian trade bookstores, wholesalers, individuals, organizations,
and educational institutions:* Please contact General Distribution Services,
325 Humber College Blvd., Toronto, Ontario, Canada M9W 7C3;
tel. Ontario and Quebec (800) 387-0141, all other provinces
(800) 387-0172; fax (416) 213-1917.

Trifolium's books may also be purchased in bulk for educational, business,
or promotional use. For information, please telephone (416) 483-7211
or write: Special Sales, Trifolium Books Inc., 250 Merton Street, Suite 203,
Toronto, Ontario, M4S 1B1

Baptism of fire, all happening within
Illusions burn like tall grass
In the wild and reckless wind
And now they're coming down around me
And I am rising up
Like a great bell resurrected
Ringing loud and true
The only way out is through

— "Baptism of Fire," Julie Snow

For Bob and Nic and Leah,
who have shared much of the journey.

CONTENTS

ACKNOWLEDGMENTS

One of the most gratifying and surprising results of having taken the step to get a cochlear implant has been meeting and corresponding with the dedicated people working in this multidisciplinary field. Surgeons, audiologists, researchers, and other professionals have been generous with their time and knowledge in helping me to ensure that this book is an accurate and useful resource. I am especially indebted to the following for reviewing my manuscript and offering corrections and suggestions: Peter Blamey Ph.D., Noel Cohen M.D., Carol De Filippo CCC-A, Ph.D., Jane Opie CCC-A, Ph.D., Julia Sarant B.Sc., Dipl. Aud., Robert Shannon Ph.D., David Shipp M.A., Aud(C), and Joanne Syrja M.P.A., H.S.A.

In addition, I thank Larry Orloff, Ellen Long, and Bena Shuster for reviewing the manuscript and offering comments, suggestions, and enthusiastic support. Esther and Jonathan Dostrovsky, good friends that they are, supplied a peaceful retreat where I could write.

But the list doesn't end there. There were many others who reviewed parts of the manuscript or gave me substantial assistance in the research and writing of this book. To them too, I am grateful: Rick Apicella Esq., Charles Berlin Ph.D., Arthur Boothroyd Ph.D., Dorothy Boothroyd-Turner M.E.D., Melissa Chaikof, Graeme M. Clark M.D., Don Eddington Ph.D., Warren Estabrooks M.Ed., Dipl. Ed. Deaf, Lisa Geier M.A., CCC-A, Susan Goldberg Ph.D., Leah S. Goodman, Linda Hanusaik M.Sc., Aud/SLP(C), Nancy Hoffmann, William House M.D., Brian Iler LL.B., Bronya Keats Ph.D., Susan Lawrence, Patricia Leake Ph.D., William Luxford M.D., Douglas P. Lynch, Louise McMorrow, Gary Malkowski, Linda Miland, Jean Moore Ph.D., Monique Moore, Marilyn Morton Dipl. Ed. Deaf, Marilyn Neault Ph.D., Julian Nedzelski M.D., Steve Otto M.A., Blake Papsin M.D., Geoff Plant TTCTD, Tilak Ratnanather Ph.D., Karen Rockow, Edwin Rubel Ph.D., Brenda Ryals Ph.D., Teri Sinopoli M.A., CCC-A, and William C. Stokoe Ph.D.

I am indebted as well to the wonderful community of cochlear implant users around the world who have shared their experiences in the pages of *CONTACT* and other journals, in correspondence, on the Internet, and in person.

I wish to thank Wendy Thomas for being such a careful and understanding editor, and Trudy Rising and Grace Deutsch of Trifolium Books Inc. for having faith in the value of my book.

And finally, I owe more thanks than I can express to my husband, Bob Biderman, for his love and support.

FOREWORD

My co-workers at the Johns Hopkins Hospital and I have long felt that it was only after we learned to listen to those who are deaf that we appreciated the implications of hearing. For all but a few, the sense of hearing has been with us since even before we were conscious of an outside world. Naturally accustomed to this stimulation, it is nearly impossible to understand life without it.

The advent of the cochlear implant has had a profound impact not only on clinical approaches to hearing loss, but also on discussions of cultural perspectives on deafness. The deepest level of understanding is perhaps available only to those who have "been there" and experienced both hearing and deafness.

A caterpillar's metamorphosis into a butterfly may seem like an elegant and even romantic transition to the outside observer. For the caterpillar, however, the experience of metamorphosis is torment. During the transformation, it temporarily goes deaf and blind, its legs fall off, and its torso splits. The result? A transition manifested in the emergence of beautiful wings.

How does this compare to the communication change produced by cochlear implantation? The metamorphosis of a silenced sensory pathway into a functional human sense requires courage to journey into an area of great uncertainty. It means remaining motivated in that uncertainty and embracing the challenge of changing the very basis for relating to the outside world.

Many Deaf individuals shun an implant as an ill-conceived attempt to achieve acceptance in the hearing world. They claim that the reality often falls short of this expectation, leaving implant recipients in a confusing middle ground between Deaf and mainstream culture. Cochlear implantation presents challenges, and an element of struggle, and it entails risk. Yet a growing number have been enticed to at least explore their candidacy for it can offer immeasurable benefit.

Deafness affects and shapes social realities. Just as deafness is a shared disability, the process of restoring the sense of hearing is both intensely personal and collaborative at the same time. The diversity of results is testimony to the critical role that the commitment of family, friends, caregivers and co-workers can play in nurturing a successful outcome with a cochlear implant.

The result? When we think about metamorphosis, we often envision a physical change that can be observed by the human eye, but Beverly Biderman's journey into deafness and back to hearing is a metamorphosis no less remarkable for being invisible. Just as the butterfly will fly into a new relationship with the world that the caterpillar could never even imagine, so those who undertake the journey into hearing may find themselves free to relate to the world and to communicate in new ways. This compelling book reminds us that what is most important in life is our connection to others.

John K. Niparko, M.D.   April, 1998
Professor of Otolaryngology
Director, The Listening Center at Johns Hopkins
Baltimore, Maryland

PROLOGUE

Imagine yourself in a room with just a few close friends you love, talking and laughing. The conversation is quick and animated. It is too swift for you to follow on their lips, too difficult for you to understand – because you are deaf. You sit in their midst with a frozen smile on your face, your cheeks aching, afraid to break the warm mood by telling them you are unable to understand. Your heart tightens and aches too. You feel angry that you are once again shut out, angry at yourself for being deaf, and at the world for expecting you not to be. Then, imagine another day, when you have a device implanted deep within your ear to help you to hear. Imagine that with it, you hear words and phrases in the air without looking for them on people's lips. You understand – not every-thing, but enough to feel a part of the group. You hear birds that were once silent, music that was once noise. Your cheeks thaw. Your heart opens up. Your anger melts, and you feel a sense of grace.

The device within my ear is a cochlear implant. For the first forty-six years of my life, it seemed that I was helpless to do anything about the progressive hereditary hearing loss that made my world increas-ingly quiet and increasingly frustrating. My moderate hearing loss in childhood became profound by the time I reached my early teens. Although I could talk, I could understand no speech at all unless I could also see it on the speaker's lips. I could not use the telephone, nor listen to the radio. The cochlear implant my surgeon inserted when I was forty-six was the first real tool that enabled me to feel less helpless, less a victim of deafness.

This device is the first successful artificial sensory organ, the result of one of the most rapid advances ever made in medical technology. For children who cannot do well with hearing aids, it is the first major development to help them communicate in the 200 years since sign language was first established.

My cochlear implant is still somewhat of a novelty: there are only about 20,000 people in the world who have one. Hearing loss, however, is the most prevalent and fastest growing disability in North America, due to the aging of the population and the increase in noise pollution.[1,2] Moreover, profound hearing loss occurs in one in 1,000 children at birth, and one in 500 by the age of five.[3] Generally, one person in ten has some sort of hearing loss, and for roughly one person in one hundred the loss is severe or profound.[4] These people could be candidates for this little-known procedure that can allow the deaf to hear birdsong, symphonies, and speech.

The idea for this book came when Larry Orloff and I were sitting around his kitchen table in Foxboro, Massachusetts, talking about the need for people to understand what it is like to hear with this relatively new device called a cochlear implant. Larry is the editor of the quarterly journal of Cochlear Implant Club International, CONTACT. He and I talked about how it would be useful to have a book that tells people what it is like to decide to get a cochlear implant, to have the surgery, to have the equipment "turned on," and to learn to hear with this electronic prosthesis. We thought there was a need for a book that would – without exaggeration, and as honestly as possible – explain these things to someone as if he or she were there in Foxboro sitting around the kitchen table with us. Both of us had met and corresponded with many people who wanted to know what it was like to have electrodes surgically embedded in our ears to give us a sensation of rich and complex sound. Later, when I started to write and started my journey back in time, I realized that not only was I writing for those deaf people who might benefit from the prosthesis (and not all can), but also for anyone interested in our ability to transform our lives. And to help both the reader and myself to understand this transformation, I have gone back to describe where I have come from: deafness. To understand the experience of hearing with a cochlear implant, you need also to understand the experience of deafness.

This book has many voices – you will hear mine, mostly, for this is above all a personal story of my experience of deafness and of hearing with a cochlear implant. You will also hear the voices of other deaf people and parents of deaf children. I have placed their quotations throughout the book in order to give you an appreciation of the huge range of responses that people have both toward deafness itself, and toward the experience of hearing with a cochlear implant. Many of these responses are very different from my own.

Some of you will be familiar with cochlear implants only as a controversial device that some deaf people do not want. I hope this book will shed light on the controversy and show that there are no prescriptions that fit all deaf people. The decision to obtain a cochlear implant is a personal one for a deaf person and parents of deaf children to make themselves. For me, in the end, my cochlear implant has allowed me to do what I want to do with far greater ease, and to do new things that give me tremendous joy. It has done no less than transformed my life.

I want to say a few words about the organization of this book. The first chapter describes my initial experiences in having my cochlear implant equipment "turned on." Nothing fully prepared me for what I encountered. The next chapter describes my roller-coaster ride in the days following, as I learned to make sense of the strange sounds my new prosthesis gave me. Chapters Three and Four go back chronologically to describe how I became deaf and adapted to deafness as I grew up, and describe the effects of deafness on my family. In Chapter Five, I discuss how I decided to get a cochlear implant, and what was involved in the testing and surgery. It is here that I describe the device, its history, how it works, who is a candidate for it, and how well it works (for both adults and children). In Chapter Six, I present the opposition of some people in the Deaf culture to this procedure and put that opposition in perspective. The final chapter of the book describes some of the shortcomings of the technology and some promising developments on the horizon. In the Epilogue, I indulge in some reflections on life post-implant. And finally, I hope that those of you who would like more information will find the annotated endnotes and the listings of resources and recommended reading at the back of the book useful.

TURN ON

What if in my waking hours a sound should ring through the silent halls of hearing? ... Would the bow-and-string tension of life snap? Would the heart, overweighted with sudden joy, stop beating for very excess of happiness?[1]
– Helen Keller

Thursday, July 8, 1993: the most anxiously awaited day of my life. Six weeks after surgery, it is "turn on" day. The incision behind my ear has healed, and I am ready to get my external equipment connected and turned on at the clinic. I ask Bob, my husband, not to come with me. The turn on will be a private moment that I just cannot contemplate sharing, even with my husband, so laden is it with a lifetime of hopes and dreams. In spite of my resolve not to expect too much, the stories about people who can understand on the telephone even on the first day have made me excited that I too might achieve wonders.

At my first meeting with my surgeon many months previously, he had suggested that my expectations would need to be modest, in view of the fact that I had been profoundly deaf for more than thirty years. My memory of sound might be poor, and considerable atrophy of my auditory system may have occurred. Not only might I not be able to understand speech better, he said, but a cochlear implant was not very helpful for hearing music. He could predict only that lipreading would almost certainly be easier, and that I would hear more environmental sounds such as birds, ambulance sirens, and honking horns.

Before that meeting with the surgeon, however, I had written a short simple list of my two priorities: to be able to understand speech better, and to enjoy music as much as I used to before it gradually faded away over the years. Much as I was habituated to my hearing aid, I did not seem to be appreciably benefitting from it. While wearing it, I could hear some environmental sounds if they were nearby, but I was unable to understand any speech unless I could also lipread. Many people with a cochlear implant, on the other hand, could. When the surgeon asked if I wanted to proceed, I found myself saying yes. I felt I had nothing much to lose, and perhaps much to gain.

When I first decided to go ahead with the surgery, I was reluctant to tell anyone other than very close family and friends. I was afraid of appearing pathetic, of seeming to be chasing cures. "What?" I could imagine people asking. "After all these years of deafness, are you still looking for a miracle? Haven't you accepted it yet?" I had invested so much time and emotional energy into adapting to my deafness since childhood that it was hard to acknowledge that yes, it was still a problem, and that I accepted it only with great reluctance. Later, I became comfortable with my decision, warning those who enthusiastically offered to phone me up and talk to me on the telephone right away after I got my implant that I couldn't expect much. But secretly, I was confident that, somehow, I would do well.

Today, I meet with David Shipp, my audiologist, for my turn on. I tell him how difficult the six-week wait since the surgery has been. David is a warm and outgoing audiologist, popular with his patients. He has published a number of research papers on the subject of predicting cochlear implant outcomes. He confides that it's always very difficult for him too, and that he is anxious to find out how well his patients will do. Audiologists and surgeons have few indicators to help them predict the ability of a patient to make good use of an implant. Duration of profound deafness (more than thirty years in my case), age at implantation (I was forty-six), and motivation (mine was excellent) are three main factors. The first two were strikes against me, but the third, my high motivation to hear, was in my favor. One researcher speculates that there is a chemical basis for the role of motivation in cochlear implant performance: motivation may release neurotransmitters that improve brain functioning![2] Even so, surprises can result from conditions that are impossible to evaluate in advance, such as the placement of the electrode array relative to surviving neurons in the ear, and the health of the central auditory system in the brain. There are probably also some mysterious factors affecting success that no one has yet completely identified.

I am lipreading David, although I also wear my old hearing aid in the ear that does not have the implant. If he turns away from me, I cannot understand a word he says. I am an excellent lipreader, and most people meeting me for the first time and chatting with me do not realize that I am deaf, and that I understand what they are saying only by watching the movements of their lips and the expressions on their faces. Lipreading is something I have picked up unconsciously and have probably been doing all my life. However, it is tremendously stressful to manage in a hearing milieu with so little sound information, relying almost exclusively on my eyes to comprehend what is being said.

Sign language was never a seriously considered option for me. When I was a child, and my hearing loss started to create problems for me in school, I already had speech, and my parents were reluctant to send me away to a residential school for the deaf. When I was an adult, still struggling with my profound hearing loss, I could have decided to use sign language as my main method of communication, but I didn't. I was too immersed in the hearing world, with a hearing husband, and a profession as a computer systems analyst that required me to work with people who knew no signs. So I continued to rely on lipreading.

For the fitting, David takes out of a box a gray digital processor the size of a cigarette package. He connects it to a cord leading to a beige microphone that curves over the top of my ear like a hearing aid. He connects this microphone to a shorter cord leading to a small one-and-a-half-inch wheel-shaped transmitter that has a magnet in its hub. When he tries to fit the wheel over the hard lump behind my ear where the implanted receiver and its magnet sit beneath my skin, it falls off. He replaces the magnet inside the wheel with a stronger one to compensate for my thick hair, and I feel it go *clunk* when he places it behind my ear. This time it stays on snugly.

He inserts my processor box in a slot in a programming device connected to his computer and settles in front of his screen. He explains that he is going to present me with a series of three tones for each electrode. I listen carefully and find that they sound like what I used to hear when I had a hearing test and could still hear the test signals. These, however, are a little more electronic sounding and harsh. The high-pitched beeps sound like whistles, the low buzzes like horns. Some people weep when they hear these beeps and buzzes after being without sound. I am calm: I have never been com-pletely without sound, and I feel that these tones are like strange cousins to sounds I've heard with hearing aids. I am to tell David when I can first hear the softest tone he presents for each electrode. From that information he will set my threshold levels.

The cochlea is like a piano: different parts of it are responsible for different pitches. Inside it, my surgeon has strung electrodes so that when they are activated, they depress different keys on my "piano." The result is that I can distinguish the pitch getting progressively higher as we go up the string, testing each electrode in turn.

In a normally hearing ear, sound enters the ear as pressure waves that make the middle ear's eardrum and small bones vibrate. These vibrations travel across the oval window of the inner ear to the fluid inside the cochlea. There, the movement of the fluid causes the tiny cilia (hairs) on the hair cells of the cochlea to bend and send electri-cal energy along the auditory nerve to the brain. A cochlear implant system, however, bypasses the outer ear, the middle ear, and the inner ear's cochlear hair cells.[3] Instead, it directly stimulates the auditory nerve fibers inside the cochlea.

While David is testing me, I can't be sure when I am hearing a faint tone and when I am imagining one in my head. Phantom sound is a problem for me. My auditory imagination has become very good over the years, especially because my hearing loss was progressive.

David checks and re-checks until he is satisfied that he has valid low thresholds. Then we repeat the test on each electrode, but this time for loudness, or "comfort" levels. I am to tell him when a tone becomes "loud but bearable." This, too, is difficult for me to gauge. How loud is too loud for someone who has had little experience with hearing? Moreover, I have the idea that a wide range between the low and high thresholds will give me more benefit, so I try to push my limits and stop only when the sound is unbearable. For the high-frequency sounds, this turns out to be when I feel a stab of pain in my head. For the low-frequency tones, it is when I feel my blood pressure rising to an uncomfortable level. This strategy is a mistake, and at every fitting session in the following weeks, I will bring those loud sounds down to a more bearable level and narrow my range. While a very narrow range is not a good idea, after a certain point, a wider range doesn't give a significant benefit. I will find that with my comfort levels too high, I flinch at some voices and sudden sounds, and need to keep the sensitivity of my processor turned down too low for the program in it to operate at its best.

We have now given my processor a "map" of the high and low thresholds for each electrode. The good news is that each of the twenty-two electrodes is functioning. In rare cases, an electrode will fail during or after surgery, or when activated, it will cause an unpleasant response such as a facial twitch. However, electrodes can be turned off (or rather, not activated at all), and turning off a few does not need to compromise performance; the audiologist can program the processor so that adjacent electrodes receive the stimulus meant for the non-functioning ones. Although multiple electrodes are better than one electrode for speech discrimination, more electrodes do not necessarily give more benefit. Some systems have sixteen electrodes, some six, and some twenty-two; some people with six electrodes may do better than some people with twenty-two.

David removes my processor from his computer and gives it to me to place in the nylon pouch looped over my skirt belt. He gives me a little pep talk about how at the beginning, some people find that voices are mechanical-sounding, like cartoon-character voices, and how others find that voices sound good almost immediately. He then turns on all the electrodes and asks, "How does that sound?" I am startled and do not realize that he is no longer simply presenting single tones to me for testing. When he had tested each electrode, they had sounded like either whistles or horns. Now, with them all turned on, I hear a cacophony of horns and whistles going off together. David's voice, when I realize it is a voice I am hearing, does not sound like Donald Duck or Mickey Mouse as David had warned it might. It sounds like Harpo Marx working his horns and whistles. I feel nauseous from the dreadfulness of the sound, and the loudness, and I can see my disappointment mirrored on David's face.

> My audiologist asked if I could hear her. After seeing me shake my head, she expressed surprise. Then, it hit me. The undulating waves I was feeling in my head were actually sounds, not my imagination.[4]
>
> – Kristin Buehl, born profoundly deaf, describing her turn-on experience at the age of twenty-one

He continues to talk, and keeps asking, plaintively, "Does it sound better now?" It doesn't. His voice is booming, and hollow and mechanical. It is full of beeps and buzzes.

Some months after my turn on, I realized that my wits alone were not going to help me succeed in this venture. While I did not feel pathetic, thanks to my small successes with my new hearing, I felt anguish that the greater successes of others seemed to be out of my reach. I wish it were not so, but even today, I feel a pang of pain when I compare myself to those who seem to be more successful in using their implants: the ones who can talk freely on the telephone to anyone, the ones who can understand announcements over raspy public address systems, the ones who seem to be only mildly hearing impaired. When you live your life in a hearing environment, deafness of any degree can be hard to bear.

David patiently walks me around the clinic to have me listen to all the torturous environmental sounds: he runs water in the sink, and it sounds like Niagara Falls (close-up); he crumples up a plastic bag, and it makes a harsh crackling sound (I thought plastic bags rustled softly in peace); he opens a door that squeaks loudly (why hasn't he oiled its hinges?). We walk down the corridor, our shoes making a tremendous clatter when they hit the floor, and I hear noisy conversations everywhere. David suggests that we go outside to listen to buses and birds and cars. He is disappointed that there is no large bus taking off outside the door. The small one idling in front of me seems loud enough. There is a confused jumble of noises, and I'm relieved when we head back inside.

We go back upstairs, and David shows me how to take care of the equipment (quite simple), and how to put it on and take it off. I need to force myself to pay attention to him, as I am already making plans to abandon it all as soon as I get home. When he has finished with his explanations, David hands the cardboard box for the equipment to me and walks me to the door. When he asks where I am parked, I lipread him and say, quickly, "I'm taking a taxi." I had been too uncertain about how I'd manage with my new hearing to drive to the hospital, and had planned to take a leisurely walk through the park and ravine to get home. Now, I just want to get home fast.

When I get outside, however, I decide to go ahead with my plan to walk. The traffic noise is loud, but understandable – what I normally hear with a hearing aid but at least ten times louder, with some interesting high-pitched sounds thrown in. I leave the hospital and cross the road to the ravine. It's gorgeous on this beautiful summer day and voluptuous with sound. There are what seem to be thousands of birds, all very noisy, but the sounds, together, are rather nice. I feel connected, a part of the scene. I throw a small stone into the stream, and the plunk is solid and recognizable. My feet scuff against the gravel path, and the sound is satisfying and pleasant. People's voices as they pass are thunderous and harsh, and I hear them approaching long before I can see them. I see a group of little children from a day camp, strung together with a rope. They are singing a song, and I can catch a rhythm to their singing, and it sounds high and sweet and fine.

After I emerge from the ravine, I stop off for an ice cream and find the store filled with whistling loud noises. I try to localize the sounds, but there are too many of them, and it's confusing. It's very hot, the hottest day of the summer, as it turns out. A few blocks later, I get a drink, and the sounds inside the coffee shop are again impossibly loud and raucous. I am amazed by how voices are carrying. I'm used to hearing voices only when people are talking directly to me, but now I can hear them from a long way off. Everything is so loud.

> When I came home from my first mapping session, I ran into the house, turned on the stereo and started dancing. Then I went to phone my parents. My father answered the phone, and I said, "Dad, this is Doug." He said, "Could you turn the stereo down?" Then it suddenly hit my father that he was talking to me on the phone, and all I could hear was sobbing.[5]
>
> – Douglas Lynch, who was profoundly deaf for fifteen months from autoimmune inner ear disease before getting an implant in 1995

I arrive home, come through the door, and trudge upstairs with heavy feet and a heavier heart, making a whistling noise at every step. My teenage son, Nic, is away at a summer camp, but Bob is upstairs at his computer. He turns excitedly to ask how it went. He can tell from my face that I am miserable. "Listen," I say, "there's something the matter with it," and I sway back and forth in the hall from one foot to another, whistling as I sway. "Oh, that," he says, relieved, "those are the floorboards creaking." I discover, for the first time, that there are loud creaking floorboards everywhere in my house. When Blossom, the dog, walks, she too makes them creak. I flirt briefly with the idea of moving to a house with concrete floors.

I had met Bob because I was deaf. We had both been at a party, where Bob, an outgoing person who likes people, had approached me to make conversation. When he asked me what my name was, I had apparently got up from my chair and walked away. His curiosity was piqued, and he asked a mutual friend why I had snubbed him (or at least, as he put it, not waited to first get to know him before snubbing him). She explained that I was deaf and probably had not heard him talking to me. When Bob asked how he could call me up to ask me out for a date, she gave him my telephone number and told him that he would need to call my mother to have her relay messages for me as I could not understand on the phone.

I keep hearing a strange whistling sound at the end of Bob's and everyone else's words. It's only after I realize these words are often plural that it occurs to me that what I am hearing must be the sibilant *s*. It is a sound I have not heard for forty years.

Like many people with a profound sensorineural hearing loss (or "nerve deafness") which is caused by problems in the auditory nerve or inner ear or both, I have a "left-corner" audiogram. The curve on the chart that displays what I can hear shows a small bulge for the bass low-frequency sounds plotted at the bottom left corner of the chart, and a deep dip for the more treble pitches plotted to the right. No matter how much my hearing aid amplified the higher pitched sounds, like the *s* sound, I was unable to hear them. With my hearing aid on, I could hear the beat of a drum, but not the high notes of a flute; the long vowel *oo*, but not the consonants *s* or *t* or *v*.

My speech, before I got my cochlear implant, sounded spongy, with the ends of words trailing off, and the consonants missing. I once met a woman who was a speech pathologist. I introduced myself, saying only, "I'm Bev." Yet a few minutes later when I explained that I was deaf, she said, "I know. I could tell from the way you pronounced your name. You just mouthed the *v*, instead of saying it." It's difficult to use sounds in your speech when you can't hear them yourself. After I began to hear with a cochlear implant, my speech improved, and my words had more shape and precision to them.

Bob and I get into my car to go on a listening trip to a pet shop and a city farm zoo. I feel like a small child on an adventure. I'm excited, and happy to be sharing this experience with him. After I put the key in the ignition, a strange whine comes on. I have never heard the warning to fasten my seatbelt before and need to ask Bob what it is. I think I can also hear a rattle under the car, but Bob is not much help in describing it. When I ask him what it sounds like, he says, "About five hundred dollars."

Inside the pet shop, I'm unable to hear the birds, because there is too much Muzak for me to hear anything but noise. The pig and rooster sounds at the zoo are fascinating, and I stare at the animals' and birds' mouths as they squeal and crow, to try to make sense of what I am hearing. Here and everywhere, I sense that I'm like an infant peering intently at faces, trying to understand what their noises and jabbering mean.

In my second coffee shop of the day, the voices, the cash register, and the clattering dishes are loud and harsh. I make the mistake of getting potato chips. Just the crackling bag is incredibly noisy, and the crunch as I chew is almost unbearable. I play with dropping the metal top from my bottle of juice, spinning it on the table over and over again to hear the intricate music it makes.

> It was a horrible experience. ... Sounds were very garbled. ... I couldn't distinguish between planes going over and people yelling. I was accustomed to a silent world. I didn't know where all this screaming was coming from.[6]
>
> – *Angela Theriault, who received an implant as a teenager*

At home, as I make dinner, our fridge sounds like a jungle – all those rustling plastic bags and rattling jars and bottles! And water running! And dishes hitting hard surfaces! I use my TTY (a keyboard telephone device that displays conversations from another TTY) to call a friend who has a cochlear implant, and ask her if it is supposed to be like this. When I tell her about the chirping whistling noises in my house, she starts to cry, misunderstanding, and insists I am hearing birds for the first time. In my fridge? She advises me to turn my sensitivity level down. This control knob causes my processor to be more or less sensitive to soft sounds. Turning it down results in my hearing less sound, and the world becomes more comfortable.

After dinner, we visit friends. They are so excited about my new hearing that they both talk at once. I can't distinguish their voices when that happens, and it's confusing. The range between the softest and loudest sounds I can hear with my implant is less than one-fifth of the range of a normal hearing person, and therefore my ability to make fine distinctions between signal and noise or foreground and background is poor. This is why background noise is so difficult for most people who wear a cochlear implant. Moreover, it will take me time to learn how to tune out noisy background sounds. For now, I am as distracted by ambient sounds as a baby or small child.

That night, after having worn my processor for more than twelve hours, I go to sleep, tired but wired and on edge. I toss and turn all night, thinking that I have made a mistake. I should have waited for the technology to mature. This device is crude. I wake up feeling grim. I find the equipment awkward to put on, and the cord hanging between my ear-level microphone and the processor on my belt is uncomfortable and tugs when I turn my head. But things sound a bit better. My brain is starting to put the beeps and buzzes together and make sense of them.

I was ten years old when I first started to wear a hearing aid. I remember being acutely embarrassed by the box that I wore in a pouch my mother had sewn on my undershirt, with the old-lady gray cord snaking up my neck to the pink button sticking out of my ear. I don't feel the embarrassment of my childhood when I again wear a cord snaking down my neck with my implant system, but the remembrance of my old discomfort is painful.

In the morning, I visit the clinic for my second fitting, and this time, I don't push the comfort level for the sounds up as high. We cut them out at a softer level. David now sounds more like Donald Duck, and less like Harpo Marx. On some easy tests he gives me, I surprise myself by doing not too badly: I can hear the *sh, s, t, f,* and *p* sounds when I'm not looking at David. I find I need to listen to these sounds, which are beginning to sound less like whistles, in order to understand speech. With my hearing aid, I had listened for the bass sounds to make sense of speech; now I am listening for the treble. Treble sounds give 95% of the information used in understanding speech. Bass sounds, while they account for 95% of the volume of speech, provide only 5% of the information used for comprehension. I feel I'm on the right road to understanding what I hear and am heartened. I even recognize one short sentence – "What's your name?" – without lipreading, when David gives me a printed list of multiple choice sentences and then says one. I leave feeling encouraged.

> So [the audiologist] covered up her mouth, and she said another word; I repeated it. She said the next word; I repeated it. I did this for four words. ... I looked at my daughter and she jumped up and she was crying, and screaming, "It's a miracle!" I looked at my wife, and she was crying. ... Then all of the sudden, all the tears flowed. ... I said to myself, "My God, it's beautiful; as rotten as it sounds, it's beautiful!"[7]
>
> *– Gil McDougald, former Yankee baseball player, recalling his turn-on experience*

The next day Bob and I go to a picnic on Toronto Island with some friends. There will be music, and I'm apprehensive. Some implantees say that music sounds like marbles rolling around in a clothes drier. Once again my friends are excited for me, and two of them present me with a wrapped gift. It is a set of tapes of nature and environmental sounds (loons and frogs, as well as buses and motorcycles). There are guitars at the picnic, and my friend Howard, a computer scientist, sings his "Mildly Luddite Love Song." I am relieved and pleased: his guitar sounds so intricate, complex, and beautiful. Before, I would have heard (and tried to enjoy) just a simple strum. It would have sounded the same if it was a washboard or a guitar. Now it sounds beautiful. Watching Howard's face, I understand his lyrics with more ease too:

> *My true love lives in Montreal.*
> *We parted there last night.*

*Some say we should telecommunicate, but we'd really rather
write.
I get E-mail, voice-mail, cellular calls and fax.
I'd rather get an old-fashioned rag paper note with a spot of
sealing wax.8*

For some time I had felt starved for music. I felt a hungering for the
swell of beautiful sounds that could fill my soul. I knew that many,
but not all, people disliked music with their cochlear implant, and I
was determined that I would be one of those who enjoyed it. One of
my major successes with my cochlear implant has been that I indeed
have come to take great joy and solace from music with it, even from
the early days. I can distinguish the melody and the emotion behind
lyrics and chords. I believe that I can take this pleasure because I had
no preconception of what perfect music is supposed to sound like.
Those who do are often disappointed.

My friends' voices are starting to sound more and more natural, and
I think I am starting to understand them better, especially in the case
of women's voices, which have less volume and blare than men's. I
hear a soft sighing noise, and notice that it dies out when the leaves
on the trees stop trembling. With Bob's help, I identify it as the
sound of the wind in the trees, a lovely sound that I can't remember
ever hearing before. It starts to rain, and we head back to the island's
ferry boat. I'm thoughtfully supplied by friends with an umbrella
and plastic bags to cover my head and equipment. In fact, except in
a downpour, my hair is sufficient to protect my headpiece, and the
processor's nylon pouch protects it when I wear it under my clothing. I'm exhausted when we get home, but happy.

I fall into a deep sleep only to be awakened in the night by
loud head noise: tinnitus.9 This is a vexing noise that afflicts
many people who have defective hearing. It can be soft or loud,
sound like running water or a hum or whine or even a roar.
Hearing people may get mild and temporary attacks after a rock
concert or a loud party, or permanent tinnitus after exposure to

On August 15, 1988, I was hooked up to my processor. That day was my thirty-third birthday, and my husband's first day of his executive MBA program. I now had the world's worst hair cut [from my implant surgery], a bunch of sounds I was trying to figure out, two young daughters, and my husband was gone for the week. I was fine with all this. I lost control when the dishwasher broke![10]

– Kay Basham

drugs or other triggering factors. The next morning, when I awake, it is still there. I feel disappointed. Perhaps I have pushed myself too much. I take it easy for the rest of the day and spend time corresponding by electronic mail with people I know around the world who have cochlear implants. They all encourage me to relax, to give it time, and to "let it happen."

The next day, Monday, I visit my dentist in the morning, and present him with a list of procedures and equipment that the device manufacturer warns I should stay away from at any medical facility: electrosurgery, diathermy, electroconvulsive therapy (hopefully not at the dentist), ionizing radiation therapy, and Magnetic Resonance Imaging (MRI). The last one, MRI, is the most dangerous procedure on the list: the imaging magnet is strong enough to dislodge my implant and cause grievous damage. (For those who know they may need MRI, there is an alternative surgical method that avoids the use of an implanted magnet.[11]) My dentist reads the warning seriously and says he will not use electrosurgical equipment to cauterize any tissue wounds, but will use other methods instead. He passes me and my list on to the young dental hygienist, who is completely bewildered about how to deal with me. She's obviously afraid that something will break. She cheers up when she is able to locate the whooshing sound for me (the suction device) and manages to clean my teeth (and remind me to floss).

I drive to my office at the university. There, I investigate where the odd sounds are coming from, and my colleague Frank joins me in the hunt. We locate the motor in the ceiling (a low rumble) and the air-conditioning outlet (a soft whistling). He confirms that yes, the *crash, slide, click,* and *thud* of the heavy crash bar doors are rather loud. He gets up on a chair to listen to the strange steady hum of my fluorescent light, which he pronounces normal. I complain that the computer sounds noisy, and he puts his ear near my computer and listens to the whirr of the fan. Also normal. Then we walk out into the hallway, where I hear a high-pitched whine. Incredibly, Frank hears nothing at first, and I need to indicate to him when it gets louder. Then he hears it, and we discover it's coming from the electrical wiring closet outside his office. Once he identifies it, he finds it annoying and gets on the phone to call the maintenance staff to get it fixed.

Conducting environmental sound hunts with a hearing person is crucial. Once I understand what a sound is, I can put it in the background and ignore it just as hearing people usually can. Moreover, the next time I hear it, I will understand what it is, and not be distracted by it. One woman I know who lives alone used to keep her implant's processor turned off when she went home because the sounds everywhere in her apartment were confusing and disturbing.

Later, I was amazed at how I had managed for most of my life with so little sound. The difference between what I hear with a cochlear implant and the low, rough sounds I heard with my hearing aid is enormous. One day, with my cochlear implant off and my hearing aid on, I listened to myself talk. The s and sh sounds felt like a fan blowing softly on my lips and tongue; I couldn't hear them. I picked up a butter knife and tapped the side of a wine glass. I heard a dull thud, which I realized originated in the vibrations I felt with my fingers holding the knife, rather than in my ear. I used to believe that this dull thud was a "clang." But when I turned my implant processor on and listened to the knife against the glass a second time, I heard a very different high-pitched spiraling sound. Moreover, I could no longer feel the vibrations in my fingers! I realized that the sound I had "heard" all those years with a hearing aid had been nowhere near being a "clang." When my hearing got progressively worse, I must have filled in the ever-enlarging blanks using my sense of touch and my auditory imagination.

I have a screen-saver program on my computer that paints across the screen beautiful sweeps of color and shape when I haven't touched my keyboard for a few minutes. Before I received my implant, I would watch those changing colors and shapes weaving and dancing on my screen and with my vivid auditory imagination I would hear a symphony in my head. I would imagine the sounds getting louder and softer, and the pitch and melody changing in time to the movement on my screen. After I got my cochlear implant, the music stopped. The implant filled my head with so much sound, that I had no need to imagine it and can no longer do so.

The next day is my sixth day since turn on. I drive to a computing conference, COMDEX Canada, counting out loud and reciting the alphabet in the car as I drive, just to hear my new sounds. At the conference, the noise level in the hallways is very high, but the lectures are enjoyable. I listen to three different speakers in ten minutes, and each has a very different quality of voice. The first has a breathy voice, the second has a deep, gruff voice, and the third, the executive vice president of Microsoft, has a clean, clear voice. I know that I am hearing more of their speech than I would have with my hearing aid. I find myself listening to words and sibilants more than to meaning. "Chips!" "Shipped!" They all whistle and ring. I scribble notes not only about the new technology they are talking about, but about mine, too. "Basses boom," I write. And: "New operating system to be shipped by Christmas." Words are so much more interesting to listen to now. "Poss-i-bil-i-ty," "Data-base-s." I fiddle with the controls on my processor, lowering and raising the sensitivity level during the lectures. I notice several people in this technical audience openly staring at my new gadget. They probably want one too.

The following day marks one week of listening with my cochlear implant. I take stock and realize the tinnitus has gone, and the severe headaches that had plagued me several times a week since my early teens have disappeared virtually overnight. I had feared that the headaches were caused by the amplification I was getting with my hearing aid, and that a cochlear implant might make them worse. However, it seems the headaches may have been caused by the huge strain of trying to make sense of speech with very little else but lipreading to guide me. I also realize that I feel more mellow and at peace with myself and the world.

It has taken me a long time to understand the anger I stored up as a result of my frustration in trying to pass as hearing with so little actual hearing. I was embarrassed by my deafness and tried to cover it up by over-achieving and bluffing, but at tremendous psychic cost. I would get angry at myself for being deaf, and at others for not understanding my unspoken communication needs. My hearing loss became profound during my preteen and teen years, when I needed to at least appear to be like everyone else. During those years, it was important to act normal, which meant hearing. Moreover, there was much more shame attached to all disabilities then than there is today. I really came to understand the magnitude of my efforts to pass as hearing, when I got more hearing and began to see how little I really had before. I was then able to forgive myself for my deafness, and forgive others for not understanding what even I had not understood.

As the weeks and months pass, I become progressively more comfortable with the new sounds, and they begin to seem more natural and meaningful. My frequent fitting sessions result in a program for my processor that does not make the sounds seem so harsh or loud. Nevertheless, by the end of my third month, to my dismay, I am still understanding little or no speech without lipreading. However, I can distinguish the components of speech, the consonants and vowels, with far greater success than with my hearing aid. I expect that improved speech comprehension without lipreading will come, but

> I also interpret in sign language at a monthly youth rally for the hearing impaired. Just think, a "deaf" person interpreting into signs with my back to the stage, i.e., I can't lip-read what they are saying on stage.[12]
>
> – cochlear implant user Cathy Este (Simon)

will be later for me than it is for most because of my long history of profound deafness.

One month after my equipment has been turned on, we are spending a glorious two weeks at a cottage on a remote island in Georgian Bay, just north of Toronto. Approaching the cottage from the road, I am surprised to hear a steady high-pitched tinkling sound. It is the sound of waves in the bay. Normally I would hear just a single wave lapping softly in front of me while standing at the shore. Now I can hear millions of waves crashing into one another all across the bay far from the shoreline. I grow fond of that constant comforting sound over the next two weeks and it resonates within me.

One day, sitting on the deck high above the beach, hearing the wind whistling through the poplars, seagulls squawking, children squealing, waves crashing, and crickets chirping, I decide to listen to all this as I would have in the past: with my hearing aid alone. I turn off my cochlear implant and slip my old hearing aid into the other ear. The joyful sounds around me become quiet, and I hear none of them.

LEARNING TO HEAR

It's not just what you're given
But what you do with what you've got.[1]
– Si Kahn

When I set about learning to hear with my cochlear implant, I paradoxically moved into a closer relationship with my deafness than I had ever had before. I never realized how deaf I was until I became more hearing. All those years of adaptation to a world gradually becoming more and more silent had left me with little awareness of what it was like to actually hear. But now, I could hear the crack in people's voices when they were upset, and I could hear the radio blaring rudely in the car stopped next to me on the road. I could hear the sound of dry leaves scampering along the pavement, and the sound of the wind in the trees. I was turned on to the world through sound.

But to really hear all these things, and more, and to be receptive to the sounds that were all around me, I needed to undo years of adaptation. I needed to stop tuning out sounds that I had heard before as just vague indistinct noise, and to listen. I needed to lessen my visual orientation to the world, and instead of hearing through my eyes, start to hear through my ear as well and to trust what my ear told me. I needed to reverse, if I could, the atrophy of the neural networks in my brain, the networks that made sense of sound and that had been receiving less and less stimulation over the years, becoming withered and sparse.

What was even more difficult for me was that I also had to manage my expectations. In order to find real pleasure in my hearing, I found that I needed to live in the moment, appreciating what I had, without constantly surveying what I still wanted. I had to look at the part of the cup that was half-full, not the part that was half-empty. These were the tasks of rehabilitation for me.

I decided that although I had a key factor, length of time profoundly deaf, working against me, I could create and encourage other factors that would work for me. I could make sure that I was literally immersed in sound. I would be in a language and sound immersion course, all my waking hours. I took a leave of absence from work so I would work only three days a week for the next three months. I would have the best of both worlds: I'd be able to practice my new hearing at work, and still have two days each week to relax and listen. I would be open to listening, go on sound hunts, and ask people to explain sounds to me. I would employ my ability to achieve closure, and accept ambiguity, putting together cues and clues to fill in a partial picture and make it whole. This was something I already excelled at: I was an old hand at adding two and two and coming up with five (or six or even eight). I was determined to work with what I had.

> My best practice came from my second grade daughter. ... When we did her weekly spelling lists she would finger-spell the letter as well as say it. I learned what letters sound like. When we did her vocabulary she would read the word and then use it in a sentence. I learned what words sounded like and began to learn sentences one at a time and each with a theme. We read together. Lots. She a page, I a page. ... It all added up to be the best therapy possible.[2]
>
> – Meri Garst, who hears with a multichannel auditory brainstem implant

My first experience with rehabilitative exercises took place long ago when I was in the third or fourth grade. My teacher had given up trying to convince my mother to move me to a residential school for the deaf. But, she insisted, a speech therapist should see me and try to do something about my imprecise, spongy speech. Some people had trouble understanding me. The speech therapist came to my class one morning and beckoned me to come outside. There was a commotion from the other children, who thought I had done something bad to warrant being pulled out of class that way. The speech therapist took me to the principal's office (there was no other place for us to meet) and sat me in front of a record player. She explained that I needed to listen to the voices on the record she was going to play so I could imitate them and learn to speak properly. She put the record on and left the room. I remember watching the record spin around and around. I could hear rough mumbling coming from it, but I did not have the slightest idea of what I was supposed to do. My speech therapy lasted for one lesson.

After my cochlear implant equipment was turned on, there was no formal rehabilitation therapy available for me at the adult clinic I attended, although there was for children at the local pediatric clinic. My audiologist pointed out that there was little proof that formal training or rehabilitation was actually helpful for adults. We discussed a paper on the subject of patient rehabilitation by Arthur Boothroyd,[3] a distinguished professor of hearing and speech sciences at the City University of New York. His paper seemed to show that adults did not benefit from formal training, and that they obtained enough practice from day-to-day living with an implant. The study described in his paper showed that successful implantees could understand speech without training, and although those with less success with their implant may have needed some training, they were unable to benefit from it.[4]

Children, however, obtained extensive therapy to help them learn to understand sounds with their implant, and because I had been deaf for so long, I did not feel my case was much different from that of a child who had become deaf after learning to speak. I theorized that my auditory memory of what things were supposed to sound like was quite poor, and that I would need to train myself almost from scratch to make the proper association between these strange sounds, and their meaning.

So began my reacquaintance with *Frog and Toad Together* and *Make Way for Ducklings.* I became a child again. I raided the children's section of my local library to take out sets of books and accompanying tapes, and I bought myself my first-ever Walkman. This was a thrilling purchase, for it meant that now I was going to listen to the radio and to tapes independently, without someone explaining to me what I was hearing. However, I needed Bob to show me how to use it: I didn't even understand that tapes needed to be rewound. I acquired a "patch cord" that plugged into the jack of my processor at one end and into the headphone jack of my Walkman at the other so I was directly connected to it. I took out a pile of children's talking books from the library. Going through each one, I would find one or two stories where the narrator's voice was clear, and there was little or no background music. Often I would need to ask Bob to listen to the tape, to tell me if it had music on it. The simple vocabulary and slow pace of children's stories were ideal for me. I would listen to the tape and read the book at the same time.

> She's like a teenager again, determined to make up for nearly a half-century of silence.[5]
>
> – *Vint Cerf, about his wife Sigrid's newfound passion for talking on the phone and listening to books on tape, after getting an implant at the age of fifty-three*

The first couple of times, it was hard to figure out what page the narrator was on. But, by the third time, I was following easily. And then, after a half-dozen times of *Make Way for Ducklings,* the sweet children's classic by Robert McCloskey, I could listen to the tape and follow it, without looking at the book. "Before you could wink an eyelash Jack, Kack, Lack, Mack, Nack, Ouack, Pack and Quack fell into line, just as they had been taught." I can't imagine any five-year-old learning to read that book for the first time feeling a greater sense of accomplishment than I did.

Did I progress from *Make Way for Ducklings?* Yes. I progressed to *Frog and Toad Together.* And *The Three Billy Goats Gruff.* After a few months, I started to borrow adult books from a service that supplied unabridged books for the blind. Although I needed to follow along with the book (for I could not take the time to reread adult books over and over), the sheer thrill of connecting sound with meaning allowed me to overlook the fact that I was taking much longer to read books than usual! I could look up from the page, and listening, catch words and phrases and whole sentences. This gave me a huge sense of accomplishment. I could see the improvements, and see that my cup was gradually becoming half-full.

I theorized that if listening to music and songs was recommended to those learning a new language, then it might be good for me too in my language immersion program. Language teachers feel that listening to songs in another language helps a student learn that language because the student is not focusing analytically on individual words, but synthetically on whole phrases and ideas. In any case, I was starved for music. So I raided the library's music racks too.

I took out every kind of music I could find. I borrowed not just music with printed lyrics on the liner notes that I could read as I listened, but opera, jazz, baroque, classical, new age, folk, flute, piano, guitar, symphonies, and concertos. I tried them all. Sometimes I would just plug myself in and listen for a few seconds and find that the music sounded awful. It would be just noise. I'd calmly take the tape out of my Walkman and try the next one in the pile. Out of twenty recordings, I might find one or two that sounded beautiful. It was worth it.

Listening to the beautiful music, I mourned for the first time what I had lost. I began to mourn on behalf of the teenage girl who had tried to listen to Peter Gunn jazz and Harry Belafonte calypso with her head on the floor inches from her record player. I remembered very clearly the sound of that imperfect music, when the music was going out of my life. I remembered the steady hum in the background coming from the motor of the cheap record player. I remembered reading the liner notes for the Harry Belafonte album to get clues about the lyrics that he was singing, and the pleasure I got then too when I did indeed associate music with meaning in the lyrics. Listening to these same scratchy Peter Gunn and Harry Belafonte records, thirty-three years later, I wept for that thirteen-year-old, and felt the frustration and despair that she had not been able to put into words for herself. Now I had the wisdom and language and compassion to feel for her what she had slowly lost those many years ago. Grieving was a belated but necessary step for me to take in order to finally accept my deafness.

The first piece of recorded music that sounded fine with my cochlear implant was Glenn Gould, pounding out "The Goldberg Variations" on the piano. That music was so exciting, so intricate. I listened to it over and over, and then moved on to other pieces played by Glenn Gould and other compositions by Bach. Baroque music, especially that of Bach, was the most pleasurable in the early months, since it was highly rhythmic and predictable. Initially, listening to just one instrument playing alone was easiest, since it was the least confusing, but I soon found symphonies and concertos wonderful too. I loved Mozart's *Eine kleine Nachtmusik.* Beethoven's crashing music, however, sounded too loud: the sudden crescendos were uncomfortable. Music that I heard directly through my patch cord was clearer than music I heard from regular speakers, through the air. I became so enraptured by music, that I found it hard to walk past a radio or tape deck without looking fondly at its output jack, suppressing an almost biological urge to plug myself in.

> Yet I could not bring myself to say to people: "Speak up, shout, for I am deaf." Alas! How could I possibly refer to the impairing of a sense which in me should be more perfectly developed than in other people?[6]
>
> – *Ludwig van Beethoven, who composed many of his greatest works of music, including the Ninth Symphony, while profoundly deaf*

I attribute my success with music in part to the fact that I had never heard perfect music, and so was not comparing the imperfect music I was hearing with my implant to some ideal music in my past. Some people who have a good memory of how music is "supposed to" sound are disappointed. Beethoven, for example, would almost certainly have been cruelly disappointed had he been able to make the leap forward in time to get a cochlear implant to give him back some version of his sorely missed hearing.

Some people, when they get their cochlear implant, may listen to old favorite selections of music; if the pieces do not sound the same, they may give up. Others persevere and accept that the music will sound different, and that they may need to experiment and try other pieces. Some even resume playing a violin or a piano or other instrument. Before I got my implant, I found rock music the most enjoyable, because of its loud bass beat. But when I started to listen to music with my implant, I didn't particularly like the sound of rock. I preferred the tenuous treble of violins to the blunt bass of drums.

I listened to the Beatles and for the first time was able to pick out their voices from the music of their instruments. I listened to Stan Rogers belting out "Northwest Passage" while following the song with the lyric sheets in front of me, just as I had with the talking books. I could hear the passion in Stan's voice, and the emotional meaning behind his song, as I never had before, even when I saw him perform in person years ago. Many songs moved me to tears.

A lot of things moved me to tears in the months following my turn on. It seemed that my emotions were often close to the surface and would come spilling out at strange times. I found some deep bass sounds disturbing. They frightened me in a way I did not understand. Some high-pitched sounds were so pretty. Some voices were unspeakably beautiful and touching. Chuckles on the phone and the radio and television warmed my heart. I realized I was responding to the emotional content of sounds, and finding there was emotion everywhere. The monochrome sounds I had heard before were now rich with color, some beautiful and some not.

Anthony Storr, in *Music and the Mind*, talks about the close link between hearing and emotions. He points out that hearing is much more closely related to emotions than vision is. If we see a wounded animal or person, he says, we are never as moved as we are if we hear the animal or person's anguished screams with our ears. He theorizes that the strong link between hearing and feeling may be related to the fact that we can hear before we can see, as the sense of hearing is developed in the womb early, before the sense of vision is formed.

One day, when I tried to check out new tapes at the library, the clerk stopped me because the computer showed that I already had twenty-six out. When I checked at home, I actually found twenty-seven! I decided I needed a new strategy. I had to get off the Library Interpol! So I ordered a set of rehabilitation videotapes from the University of Utah.[7] These tapes were developed at the university's medical center for the center's implant clients to use at home, because many of them lived far from the hospital. The first tapes were too easy ("Listen to the sound of the ice cubes dropping into the glass"), but the later tapes in the series of six were more challenging. The narrator gave a brief explanation of how things sound (for example, how explosive *ch* and *p* sounds were of shorter duration than the continuant consonants *sh* and *v*). He or she would then drill me by asking me to select which word was being spoken from a set of word choices displayed on the screen. "Oh," I would tell myself, "so that's how the letter *k* sounds at the end of a word." And – "Oh, that's the way the word 'book' sounds." And I would find myself squirreling away this new information, hopefully to recall it later on the fly.

I took some music appreciation courses, one of which was with a private music tutor. When I met Art Levine for the first time, I tried to explain a bit to him about my strange way of hearing, and how I didn't hear what he heard. He was unruffled. "Nobody hears the way I hear," he said. "What we hear depends on experience, memory, lots of factors we don't understand." Then he showed me a piece

> I immediately started to work on hearing the piano again. Each week, I heard more notes until I could hear the whole keyboard. I then started to teach myself to differentiate between intervals and to work on nuance and dynamics. I don't hear music as well as I did in college, but I hear a much better quality of sound with the implant than I did during the seven years I was going deaf. I can go to concerts, music workshops, and recitals really enjoying what I hear.[8]
> – *piano teacher Kay Basham*

of sheet music and, stabbing his finger at the page, said, "I hear that. When I read it, I hear it in my head. Music is mostly in our minds."

We do hear with our brains – or at least, we are supposed to. But deafness causes changes in the brain. Many studies of kittens, monkeys, and mice have shown changes in their brains caused by deafness. Deafness seemed to cause the neural pathways in the central auditory system of their brains to fail to develop properly, to degenerate, and to reorganize around the information actually getting through.[9,10,11]

These neural pathways help the brain to process and interpret sound sent to it from the ear. My neural pathways, instead of being dense with tendrils and connections as they are in people who hear normally, had likely become sparse. Some connections may have withered away or become ineffective through disuse.[12] Moreover, the auditory cortex in my brain may have become reorganized around the few low-frequency sounds I was still able to hear. If so, this adaptation of my brain might now be working against me and causing me to find basses booming and deep pitches overpowering.[13]

Similar abnormalities had probably occurred in my cochlea. The spiral ganglion cells in the inner ear that relay signals from the inner ear to the brain by way of the auditory nerve decrease in number after a period of deafness. Researchers have seen this in postmortem studies when they actually counted the number of surviving spiral ganglion cells in the inner ears of deaf people.[14] I likely had not only a weaker central auditory system in my brain, organized around a few low-frequency sounds, but also fewer spiral ganglion cells in my ear to actually transmit sound.

Strangely, researchers have not found any connection between the number of spiral ganglion cells surviving in the inner ear after death and post-implant success.[15] This seems to indicate the importance of the higher processing centers in the brain in determining how well we hear. These weak neural pathways might be at least partly responsible for the difficulty I was having in making sense of the sounds, and at least partly explain the large variations in how well people do with their implants.

But our brains are plastic, and changes do take place over time. Children generally seem to take longer to show improvements with their implants than adults do; children who were born deaf may take longer to improve than those who become deaf after birth.[16] It is possible, however, for children who are born deaf to catch up with those who became deaf after birth (but before they learned speech), as long as they receive an implant early.[17,18] Adults who have been profoundly deaf for a long period of time do not seem to do as well, at least initially, with their implants as those who have been deaf for only a short time. It is possible, however, for adults who once could hear but have been deaf for a long time to eventually catch up with those who have been deaf for shorter periods of time.[19] Researchers, looking at these improvements over time, take them to indicate that the developing system is capable of remarkable flexibility or "plasticity," and that there is substantial plasticity even in the auditory systems of adults.

Patricia Leake and her co-workers[20] found that in cats deafened at birth, the atrophy of the spiral ganglion cells in the cochlea was arrested by a course of electrical stimulation. The electrical stimulation seemed to have other benefits, too – the degeneration of the auditory pathways in the central nervous system normally caused by deafness was slightly lessened or reversed.[21] Another study by researchers in Japan measured brain activity using Positron emission computer tomography (PET) in adults who had received a cochlear implant.[22] The PET scans showed that the longer the duration of deafness was, the lower the measurable activity in the auditory cortex. Following implantation, however, they found a remarkable change in activity levels: they returned to near normal. All this evidence of auditory system plasticity gave me hope. I took heart and told people I was growing stronger neural pathways even as I was listening to *Make Way for Ducklings*.

My expectations, however, continued to be a problem. By actively working at learning to hear, I was setting myself up for disappointment, in a sense, because there was no guarantee that my efforts would be rewarded by proportionately better understanding of what I heard. When I seemed to reach a plateau, but still relied on lipreading, I became depressed. Bob tried to remind me of how far I had come since getting my implant, but he was often unable to console me. At a certain point, my rehabilitation "work" seemed to be of no avail and, rather than giving me a positive feeling about my prowess, made me feel more depressed about what I could not understand.

Deep inside, unknown even to myself until then, had been growing slowly and quietly the hope that I would achieve the miraculous, and understand easily on the phone, and understand people without lipreading, and become more like a hearing person than the deaf person I was. I could not admit it to myself, this hope, before I underwent surgery. I couldn't even admit it to myself in the first few weeks or months afterward when I was sometimes overwhelmed with disappointment about what I was hearing. But gradually, I had to acknowledge that the bitter taste in my mouth when I heard the loud strange sounds of speech but did not comprehend them except through my eyes was from the disappointment of remaining, after all, deaf.

I obsessed about the half of the cup that was still empty. I analyzed what was wrong with my implant ("basses boomed too much"). I analyzed what was wrong with the electrode array in my ear ("it's responding too slowly, sounds are bleeding into one another"). I am a computing systems analyst by profession and accustomed to solving problems by analyzing them, breaking them down into their component parts, and coming up with a solution. But this problem, of hearing with my new device, was proving to be a tremendously difficult one to solve. I decided that the biological limitations of my ear and brain, and the technological limitations of my device had finally met each other, been introduced, and were sitting down in a stalemate. I glumly decided that being able to follow *Make Way for Ducklings* was no big achievement after all. I wanted to be able to hear and understand everyone at meetings at work, even when I wasn't looking at their faces. I wanted to be able to talk on the phone to everyone. I wanted to be more hearing-like. It's hard to be deaf in a hearing world, and even harder to be given a taste of hearing and not want more. It has been said that joy lies in the freedom from all expectations. If so, then joy in my imperfect, newfound hearing meant letting go of expectations. It meant "letting it happen." I was having trouble with that idea.

I was constantly asking my family and friends to explain the mystifying sounds I heard, and sometimes I would complain to Bob that his voice was uncomfortably deep. There wasn't much poor Bob could do about that, although later, when I first tried to use the phone, he spoke in a falsetto voice a few times to help me understand him! At work, I was preoccupied with my new hearing, and at meetings, I would analyze not what people were saying, but how they said it. I would marvel at the tone of their voices, at the way they pronounced words precisely. I would make discoveries such as that the letter *t* in the word "often" wasn't silent after all. But if I was tired, some sounds were stressful. I recall once, a few days after I returned to work, a colleague asked if I had received a report she had sent. I told her that I had, but the rustling of the paper when I read it was too loud, and so I had abandoned it!

> I am often asked which particular sounds made an impact on me after the "Switch On." It may seem strange, but for the first time in five years I was aware of silence. Without my hearing I had never been sure when I was in a quiet situation. Now, I really enjoy peace and calm.[23]
>
> – *cochlear implant user Jane Shaw, Yorkshire, England*

I was having an enormous amount of difficulty breaking away from my visual orientation too. I found myself thinking that I could not possibly understand speech without seeing a person's face. I just could not trust what I heard. If I could see just a slice of the face, however – a chin, a nose, a cheek – amazingly, I would often hear and understand. Obviously there was something more than hearing at work here; my visual and hearing senses had become accustomed to working together.

It seemed that all my successful adaptations to deafness, my strategies for dealing with it, my visual orientation, conspired against my understanding speech with my new prosthesis. Oliver Sacks, writing about Virgil, a man who after almost a lifetime of blindness had his vision restored, says that Virgil could not "see" a building when he first stood in front of one.[24] It was only after he held a toy building in his hand and felt its form with his fingers while looking up at it that he could actually see the building and understand what he was looking at. So too, the sensation of sound alone was not enough for me, and my brain had to somehow understand those sounds and attach meaning to them. Usually that meant bridging sound to meaning using my visual sense, just as Virgil used his sense of touch to bridge vision to meaning.

The senses do seem to go together. When I would get a new map or fitting at the clinic (which was every few months in the first couple of years), and things sounded different, things around me looked different, too. The trees would be a brighter green, the sky a more vivid blue, the textures of things would be stronger. The world around me would come into sharper focus. It was as if accentuating my hearing accentuated my other senses too.

It is quite possible that my reliance on vision had a biological counterpart. Senses that are used more seem to develop stronger corresponding areas in the brain. There have been many studies of this plasticity in animal and human brains. For example, in one study, scientists in a laboratory trained monkeys to discriminate between sounds with slightly different frequencies. At the end of the training period, the scientists found remarkable changes in the monkeys' brains. Their auditory cortices had actually reorganized around the frequencies they had been trained on.[25] The areas in the auditory cortex corresponding to the frequencies used in the training exercises had enlarged relative to their size in untrained primates. Similarly, the reading fingers of blind people who read Braille have an exceptionally large representation in the tactile part of the brain.[26] Moreover, the part of the brain that normally handles visual stimuli may be re-wired in blind Braille-readers to process information coming from their fingertips.[27]

Perhaps the portions of my brain responsible for the processing of visual stimuli had become unusually strong. If so, the same plasticity that made my visual sense stronger in an attempt to compensate for my deafness might also work in the reverse direction. It might allow my auditory sense to grow stronger with use. And, if my auditory cortex had rearranged around the meager low-frequency sounds that I was previously getting, perhaps it would rearrange itself yet again around the rich feast of sensations I was now sending it. Or so I hoped.

But it would probably help for me to be actively involved in my rehabilitation "training" as I called the exercises I set for myself listening to talking books and music, and the sounds around me. In one of the studies in which scientists trained primates to discriminate between sounds with slightly different frequencies,[28] passive experience had far less effect on their brains than active training. When the scientists stimulated the primates with specific frequencies without expecting them to make any choices, there was a much smaller effect on the animals' brains than when they needed to actively discriminate frequencies.[29] So much for my feeble plan, which I never carried out, to train myself by listening to talking books in my sleep!

For now, I still needed to see at least a part of a face when listening to people, I needed to look at the lyrics while listening to a song, I needed to see where a sound was coming from before I could understand it the first few times I heard it. For some people, especially those who had been deaf for only a few years or less, the implant gave them enough sound information that they could make sense of speech and telephone conversations even on the day their implant was turned on. They could reach back into their auditory memory and pull out what they needed to make the proper connections. But in my case, the sounds in themselves were just not enough.

On the telephone, when I started to use it after about six months, I found myself unable to trust what I heard with my ears. People would say, "Thanks, Bev." I would respond, "Thanks, Bev." They'd say, "How is Tuesday for lunch?" I would say, "How is Tuesday for lunch?" Talking on the telephone seemed like a drill to me, and I needed to repeat what I heard to confirm that I had understood correctly. I just couldn't relax, let it happen (whatever "it" was), and trust myself to go with the flow of conversation.

I started to become increasingly critical of the sounds I was hearing. In the first few months following my turn on, my criticisms of the sounds had been helpful in adjusting and fine-tuning my processor's map. I would point out to David, my audiologist, that the "basses boomed" and we would soften them. I would point out that I had to keep my sensitivity knob turned down too low, and we would soften all the sounds across the board so I could turn up my sensitivity knob to an appropriate level. But then we reached a point where there seemed to be no more fine-tuning tricks left in David's bag, and I had to simply work with what I had.

Perfectionist that I am, I had trouble sleeping because I would rack my brains during the night to figure out why I couldn't hear better and to think of what I could do that might help. I would go into work in the morning with black circles under my eyes. I was in such a fog that I once showed up at work wearing two left shoes – and didn't realize it until noon.

It was difficult for me to move ahead in learning to hear while I was feeling negatively about the sounds I was hearing. Sometimes I even found myself lapsing back completely into my old mode of coping, and not listening at all, but simply alternating between lipreading and tuning out. I found myself recoiling from some of the sounds and criticizing their loudness and quality and clarity. So too, Oliver Sacks's Virgil, whose vision had been restored, rejected the images he was seeing with his eyes. He began to turn out the light and look away from the mirror when he was shaving himself. Eventually, unable to cope with his new vision and to make enough sense of it, Virgil grew gravely ill and lapsed back into blindness.

It seemed that the fabric I had woven of my life had become unraveled. In those months following my turn on, I had an overwhelming feeling of things falling apart. It seemed too that my balance was upset, and my carefully constructed adaptations to

For I am now, after forty years of what we will term silence, so accommodated to it (like a hermit-crab to its shell) that were the faculty of hearing restored to me tomorrow it would appear an affliction rather than a benefit.[30]

– deaf British poet David Wright

deafness had been torn down. I felt thrown back into a state like that which I must have experienced as a child with gradually worsening hearing. I was in despair, and felt helpless to do anything about it. I could not go back to my previous deaf condition, having tasted so much hearing, but I could not move ahead either. In some quiet, calm moments, I felt, quite simply, that I wanted to die. I felt this not with passion, but dispassionately, almost rationally. I wanted to peacefully slip away from the raucousness, the striving to understand, and even the small successes. I could confide this despair to no one, not even to Bob, because it frightened me, and my apparent seriousness and lack of emotion frightened me even more.

Oliver Sacks seems to be describing my own experience of things falling apart when he says: "Perceptual-cognitive processes, while physiological, are also personal – it is not a world which one perceives or constructs but one's own world – and they lead to, are linked to, a perceptual self with a will, an orientation, and a style of its own. This perceptual self may also collapse with the collapse of perceptual systems and alter the orientation and the very identity of the individual."[31]

I did not understand then, in the months following my turn on, what Sacks is describing; that understanding only came much later. However, I did realize that in order to move beyond my despair, I needed to accept the sounds I was hearing and find joy in them.

One change that helped me accomplish this was that I had the settings for my processor's map made much softer and more comfortable. Another event that helped was a series of formal rehabilitation exercises at my implant clinic. Six months after I received my implant, my clinic, now aware that rehabilitation especially for those long-time deafened like me was needed, was ready to proceed with a program of auditory rehabilitation for its clients.[32] My therapist, Linda Hanusaik, gave me a variety of practice exercises. We went through word lists to see if I could distinguish (without lipreading) between words with different consonants ("tab," "tap," "tack"), and words with different vowels ("hood," "hid," "heed"). She would introduce a set of sentences by saying, "We're going to talk about the weather" and then present sentences to me, one by one on that topic. I would try to repeat as much of each sentence as I could understand, and she would encourage me by telling me that I had "got some of it," or "got most of it" or "got all of it." She asked me to bring in magazine articles that interested me, and she would read them slowly to me. I would track her speech by repeating back what she said after each short segment or sentence.

If I squeezed my eyes shut and concentrated hard, I could understand her and repeat whole sentences quite successfully. I was drained emotionally and physically after these sessions, but exhilarated and inspired too. It was exciting to see how much I could comprehend without using my eyes. The exercises gave me the confidence to pay attention to what I was hearing and to persevere. Slowly, my attitude toward my hearing prowess turned around, and I started to again feel positive about my successes, and to accept the sounds I was hearing. My skills improved, and I started to relax and enjoy the sounds.

> At some point in time, the implant and what it can do for you normalize, just like hearing aids did. You become very familiar with what works and what doesn't work, and you start to develop other coping strategies like you did with the hearing aid. ... You eventually do not know how you are doing what you are doing – is it from listening and hearing with the implant? Or did I unconsciously pick up some visual situational or environmental cue?[33]
>
> – *Ruth Oosterhof, who has over ten years of experience with a cochlear implant*

Pat Clickener, who hears with a cochlear implant, says, "The benefit of an implant is not in hearing *per se*, but in what you can do and how you feel because you hear."[34] Rehabilitative "work" helped me to really see how much I could do and made me feel very good about what I could both hear and understand. I also felt I had some control over my progress, and that I was actively engaged in learning to hear. I could see how far I had come from the buzzes and whistles of turn-on day, and it was enormously gratifying. Certainly by actively engaging in my own rehabilitation, I was giving myself a wonderful feeling of empowerment. And the formal structured rehabilitation with a therapist reminded me repeatedly and irrefutably of my successes, large and small.

I found that with hearing, the world seemed like a less hostile place. People seemed kinder, more caring. Suddenly when I started to understand a bit of speech without lipreading, I would catch people saying "Have a nice day." They would say it to me in the store when I was looking down to put my change in my wallet. Or they would say it as I turned my back and walked away from them. Or they would say, "It's a beautiful day today, isn't it?" while I was looking away from them. I would never have caught those pleasantries before. I understood them now and felt a sense of warmth and comfort from them that I did not have when I heard nothing unless I was looking for it. These found seconds of comfort were lovely.

By one year, I was picking out phrases and sentences on the radio news, something I have no memory of ever being able to do. I also started to use the phone regularly, even at work, and began to have some good long conversations with friends and family who were willing to speak slowly. Now, five years after getting my implant, although I still cannot use the telephone as freely and easily as I would like to, my performance is average for implant users at five years. In standard tests of recorded sentences, I get from 60% to 90% of the key words and phrases in those sentences, without lipreading, depending on the test.[35] My score on standard single-syllable words (words such as "rain" and "book") without lipreading is around 30%. These words are very hard for me to understand in a test, because there are no contextual clues that another syllable in the word, or another word in a sentence might give me. My scores for these tests with my hearing aid had been zero.

A few months after my turn on, I visited a friend whom I hadn't seen since before I got my implant. She exclaimed over the huge change in me. (I found it unflattering, somehow, to hear this: wasn't I all right before?) She said I was obviously not working at hearing her as much as before, and not leaning forward in my chair. She said I didn't have the same strained expression on my face and seemed more relaxed. My speech was more distinct, she said. And – I was easier to talk to because she did not have to project as much or talk as loudly or slowly. I was thrilled by this confirmation from outer appearances of the changes I felt within.

Although there may be some disagreement about the value of therapy for adults, and indeed many adults do not get any formal therapy after receiving their implant, most audiologists would say that all children who get a cochlear implant need formal therapy of some sort to help them learn to listen and speak.[36] Audiologists usually advise parents to immerse their child in an oral program so as to get as much exposure to spoken language as possible after getting an implant.[37] However, if the child simply cannot learn to function by means of oral communication alone, then most professionals would suggest the addition of sign language to oral (spoken) communication in order that the child not be bereft of any useful means of communication. In fact, although oral communication has long been pitted against sign language communication – often in emotional, either-or terms – sign language in itself need not be a barrier to the development of oral language skills.[38]

One form of therapy used for children with cochlear implants is called auditory-verbal therapy. This therapy is used also for children with hearing aids. The therapy teaches children to listen and to make listening a part of their personalities. Learning about the world through their ears becomes second nature. The children may pick up lipreading on their own, as I did, and use their eyes to fill in some gaps, but they will not be taught to watch lips. They will be taught to use their hearing. In formal auditory-verbal therapy, a parent or other caregiver is part of each therapy session, and the therapist teaches the adult right along with the child. The therapist shows the parent or other caregiver how to help the child to hear and listen.

Practitioners such as Warren Estabrooks in Toronto steer away from old-fashioned "drill" work and turn the therapy (which is never called "training," but "therapy") into play. Estabrooks takes babies a few months old who have just been diagnosed as deaf and stays with them for several years. He engrosses the child in play with his warm personality and his impressive collection of eye-catching toys (which also keep the eyes of the child away from Estabrooks's mouth while he is speaking). He takes a bright red toy bus, for example, and playfully moves it along the table, charming the child and talking to her all the while, naming the bus, and talking about what the toy is doing. In the case of older children, he engages them in verbal repartee to help them to learn how to participate in social give and take: answering questions, discussing issues, and making jokes. He says it's wonderful when children get to the stage when they can argue with him![39]

A major goal of the Auditory-Verbal Approach (practitioners capitalize the term) is that deaf children will be completely in the mainstream in their neighborhood school and able to converse easily, as Estabrooks puts it, with the butcher, the baker, and the candlestick maker. In fact, many children with cochlear implants do achieve this goal. The therapy, however, takes a large commitment on the part of the family.

The Chaikof family of Atlanta, Georgia, is a case in point. The oldest child, Rachel, was born in 1987 with a severe-to-profound hearing loss, which became total by the time she was eighteen months old. The youngest, Jessica, was born with no measurable hearing in 1995. The girls appear to have a genetic abnormality (Waardenberg's syndrome) that may manifest in a white patch of hair, differently colored eyes, or deafness. Rachel, now a mischievous-looking nine-year-old girl with a large mop of dark curls, received her implant at the New York University Medical Center at the age of two and a half, and Jessica, the baby in the family, received hers at the same clinic at the unusually early age of fifteen months.

Fortunately for Melissa Chaikof, their mother, she is not tied up with therapy for both girls at the same time. Rachel "graduated" from auditory-verbal therapy in 1996 and now receives a checkup only once a month. Jessica recently began therapy just before she reached two years of age. She sits down with her mother five times a week and with a therapist once a week for one hour of play – and learning to listen. Melissa needs only to say, "It's time to listen," and Jessica will happily try to climb into her chair at the table.

The immersion in sound and speech does not stop with the lessons at the table: Melissa gives Jessica (and her sister Rachel) informal therapy throughout the day. She talks to them as much as possible, in a natural way as she changes the baby's diaper, for example, or helps Rachel with her homework. Melissa sometimes forgoes the use of the family's dishwasher so she and her older daughter can wash and dry the dishes at the sink side-by-side, talking as they work. The baby, Jessica, sometimes continues her formal lessons on her own. Jessica has a bead maze toy that she and her mother use at the table for speech familiarization, saying sounds as they push the beads along the maze. Later, after Melissa puts the toy back on the floor in the sunroom, she may hear Jessica happily pushing the beads along while making the sounds she heard her mother make. Although born deaf, Jessica is learning to listen and to reproduce the sounds she hears.

Our daughter is growing up knowing first-hand the richness of spoken language, learning its subtle shades of meaning and the fun of puns and rhymes. She hears birds singing and the sound of laughter. What more could we ask?[40]

– *Jane Meador, mother of Paige, who became profoundly deaf at one, and received an implant at three*

When I met Jessica shortly after she turned two, she seemed like a happy child and was babbling almost constantly. She seemed to understand everything her mother said to her, plopping down on the floor obligingly when asked to sit down, reaching for her cup when asked if she wanted more milk, and determinedly waddling off in search of her older sister when she was asked "Where's Rachel?"

Rachel's speech was fairly clear, and she seemed to be well integrated socially with the hearing children I saw her playing with. Her mother told me that Rachel can chat on the phone with her friends with little difficulty. She attends a regular school, in a class of hearing children, where the results of her language tests are age appropriate or better in all areas but vocabulary and auditory sequential memory.[41] (My own auditory memory is also poor. When people spell out a word for me, for example, I forget the first four letters by the time they get to the fifth!)

I suspect that Melissa's daughters appreciate the one-on-one time they have with their mother, and the undivided attention and praise they get during these sessions. Most of the children I have met who get auditory-verbal therapy seem to have a positive sense of their selves. None of the children are trying to pass as hearing as I did when I was a child. None of them are coping with their deafness entirely on their own. Their disability is addressed head-on with therapy and practical help in a positive way that can leave the child feeling empowered and cared for rather than disempowered and neglected.

Jessica, Rachel, and I are demonstrating the incredible flexibility of the human organism, and our ability to work, even thrive, with what we have. Just as I did with my own auditory rehabilitation after I got my cochlear implant, these children are learning each day what they can do with what they have and how far a little hearing can go.

3

GROWING INTO DEAFNESS

*The best that can be said for deafness is that it's
an invisible handicap. The worst, that it puts adults
at the mercy of their hearing children, at the mercy
of [their hearing] parents, at almost everyone's
mercy. It is one of the cruelest and most deceptive of
afflictions. It can emasculate men and devastate
women. It is an impairment of communication. But
it's not just the disfigurement of words and it's
not just broken ears. It's most often a
barrier between person and person.[1]*
– Lou Ann Walker

Most of the childhood pictures of me show a sweet-looking girl with bandages on her knees, a dog at her side, and her head cast down. I developed a way of looking down when I did not want to understand what was being said. Looking down, I understood almost nothing of what I heard. One of my earliest memories is of my mother telling me "Look up, look up when I'm talking to you." I remember the feeling of my chin pressing on my chest, and my reluctance to look up for fear of what I would hear there.

And my speech was sweet too: I used to say "bat" instead of "what" and my family found that funny. "Bevy," they'd call me from

41

downstairs. "Bat," I would say from upstairs, in the days when I could still hear my name being called from outside my line of vision. This was when I was a toddler and could not go far away. When I started to go farther, pedaling furiously on my red tricycle with my collie dog Laddie galloping along beside me, I was not as easy to call back. It was then, when I kept pedaling and pedaling, going farther and farther away from her in spite of her calls, that my mother realized that I could not hear properly. But there was an even earlier time when she realized my secret, that I was deaf.

> *My eyes are squeezed shut, and I can feel tears streaming from one eye. I am sitting on the couch in our living room, to which my older sister, Leah, has guided me. Leah, who is about eleven, is reassuring my mother. My sister is panicky, but my mother is worse – hysterical, distraught, inconsolable. I can tell somehow, maybe because I've opened my eyes briefly, that my sister is saying, "Don't worry, Mom, it's probably wax. Her ears are probably stuffed up with wax." But my mother is cry- ing. And in between her sobs, through my almost closed eyes, I can understand her say: "She's deaf. No, she's deaf. She's deaf like her father." A nail clipping had flown into my eye while my sister had been cutting my fingernails, and with my eyes clenched shut, I couldn't understand what she said when she tried to speak to me, because even at the age of four, I needed to lipread. I feel shame at being discovered, and feel I've let them down terribly.*

All the clues to my deafness were there. My father, after all, was deaf and could hear nothing except the stamp of feet that we sometimes used to call him. So had his mother been deaf, and a brother, and a sister, and other relatives whom he had left behind in his *shtetl* (Jewish village) in Russia. They were all carriers of a dominant gene for deafness that meant there was a 50% chance their offspring would also be deaf.

My father arrived in Canada by boat, at the age of sixteen, with one of his older brothers. My grandfather had come ahead, and when he earned enough money, he had sent for them. My father's mother stayed behind, and died in Russia a few years later. He lost track of the rest of his family. When he arrived, my father was faced with the challenge of learning a new language, finding a job, and settling in, with almost no hearing. But he managed, and did all those things, and did well in business as a scrap metal dealer. Following in an innocuous fashion the tradition of those in the *shtetl* to marry within their larger family (sometimes with unfortunate genetic results), he courted and then married my mother. My mother's mother had married my father's father after both older people had become widowed. My father and mother were actually stepbrother and stepsister to each other before they married. My mother, who had been born in Toronto, had normal hearing.

My father wore no hearing aids and used no sign language. He lipread. His hearing loss had gradually become profound after he learned speech in Russia, and in his new country, he was able to speak reasonably clearly, albeit in heavily accented English. With the helping ears of others, he managed quite well. Not only did my mother make and accept phone calls for him, but my father also employed a truck driver to drive him around (for my father wrongly feared that it was not safe for him to drive his truck). The driver doubled as an interpreter when needed, and he would be dragged in reluctantly to explain to my father with exaggerated mouth movements how much money a seller wanted for the scrap metal my father wanted to buy.

Although it was not noticed until I was about four, when the flying nail clipping gave me away, I may have had some hearing impairment from birth. Today, a number of sophisticated tests can be performed on newborn babies to determine if there is a hearing loss, but in 1946 when I was born, they were not available. My parents, when they realized they had lost their fifty-fifty gamble with hereditary deafness (my older sister and brother were both hearing), seemed resigned, although I know my mother also felt guilty for having taken the chance. When I was an adolescent, she pointed out to me that there were people in my father's family who had forgone parenthood in order not to risk having a deaf child. She told me sadly that they were critical of her for not doing the same. I was never in doubt, however, that she loved me very much and was glad that she had had me. Later, though, I was to decline the gamble, and chose to adopt my own son.

After the second or third grade at school, I started to get into trouble and seemed to spend a lot of time in detention or out in the hall. I was disruptive (because I did not hear what I was disrupting), and noisy (because I could not monitor the loudness of my voice). My behavior in some cases was inappropriate (because I could not pick up subtle conversational cues or follow fast-paced conversations). If my parents told my teachers that I had poor hearing (and I'm not even sure that they did), the teachers didn't do anything about it. I don't recall even having a front seat in class until the fifth grade, after I started to go to Toronto for hearing tests. Academically, I was doing poorly. Socially, I was doing even worse.

Recess time in the school playground was an ordeal. All the games the little girls my age played seemed to require hearing. There was the chanting for skipping games, especially double Dutch, that made me hold back for fear that I would not jump in (or out) at the right point. There were the elastic rope games, where the others dipped their toes over and under and between the elastics, all the while reciting some nonsense verse that I could only mutter indistinctly, praying that nobody would realize I had heard it hopelessly wrong. ("Yogi in the kaiser?") Then there were the folding-paper games, where the other girl chattered as she opened the folded paper onto little printed messages while I was supposed to look at the folds. I didn't understand these games either, for I could look at the paper the girl was wiggling in her hand, or I could watch her face and understand what she was saying, but not both. String games were also frustrating. I would watch the string figure weave on my friend's hands and understand not a word of the explanations for how to construct them.

And there were the indoor party games. I had managed to join a

club of little girls, called "The Beavers."
One of the club's favorite games was
called "Broken Telephone." We would sit
cross-legged on the floor in a circle, and
whisper into the ear of the next child a
message to be passed around the circle. I
would wait anxiously for the whisper to
reach me, and when it did, not understanding it, I would quickly make up
something to whisper into the ear of the
next girl. When the message had made
the rounds of the circle, and the last girl
to receive it announced what it was, everyone but me would be
astonished by how much the original message had changed!

> I have hollowed out the padding in my helmet and wear the [implant's] processor in hockey games. I can now hear the whistle instead of barging around until someone stops me or I notice that everyone else is stopped.[2]
>
> – *Bill Boyle*

After I started to have real problems in school, my parents asked
our family doctor what to do. We lived in the small town of Picton
on the edge of Lake Ontario, and the doctor suggested a trip to a
specialist in the city. So, when I was about ten, we started to see a
prominent ear, nose, and throat specialist in Toronto. He gave me
some tests, then had my tonsils and adenoids removed to see if they
were affecting my hearing. After the surgery, when he realized that it
had had no effect, he diagnosed a hereditary sensorineural hearing
loss and could do nothing more.

I remember the doctor putting his hand sympathetically on my
mother's shoulder when he told her there was nothing he could do.
Watching them, and the expressions on their faces, I remember feeling that I was a source of great sadness and disappointment to them
both. Then he relegated us to the basement, where his niece dispensed hearing aids. The basement had a smell of failure pervading
it. The main floor, where the doctors in white coats moved about
briskly, had been bright, exciting, and full of hope. The dim basement was none of these things.

Before sending us down to the basement, the doctor had mut-
tered something about how he had reservations about hearing aids
because eventually they could damage the hearing that was left. But,

he told us, we really had no choice. At the time, we could make no sense of his concerns. Now I realize that over the years, my hearing aid had been bombarding my ears with high sound pressure levels that may have put me at risk of losing even more hearing than I would normally have lost.[3]

The hearing aid the doctor's niece fitted me with in 1956 had a cord running from my earpiece to a box the size of a cigarette package, much like my cochlear implant processor.[4] I wore this kind of bulky aid until my early twenties when small behind-the-ear aids became powerful enough for me to use. The first thing I remember noticing when I started wearing a hearing aid was that the hearing-aid dispenser's high heels on the hard tiled floor sounded loud and piercing. Thirty-five years later when my cochlear implant was first turned on, clattering footsteps also sounded terribly loud. Unlike a cochlear implant, which gave me a whole new set of sounds to hear, however, my hearing aid merely amplified everything on the chance that my remaining hearing might pick up some of the loud sounds. (Modern aids amplify sounds more selectively.) But, for some sounds, my remaining hearing was so poor, or even nonexistent, that no amount of amplification could help.[5]

I do not remember the joy of hearing with a hearing aid. I do remember the sore, occasionally bloody ears I sometimes got from my plastic ear mould that needed to fit tightly to avoid any leakage of sound. If there was a leakage, the sound was fed back into my hearing aid, resulting in a continuous high-pitched feedback squeal. Everyone else (except knowing family members) would hold their hands over their ears and look up at the ceiling to try to locate the strange noise. But I would not hear it even though it was coming out of my own ears. I also remember the discomfort of the beige cord snaking down my neck under my clothing to the box I wore in a pocket in my undershirt (and then later in my brassiere between my breasts, where it eventually caused a bone spur). And the pink button sticking out of my ear. My mother, wanting to make things easier for me, encouraged me to cover it all with long hair and high-necked sweaters.

I adapted to wearing my hearing aid to the point where I felt lost and disoriented without it, just as those who wear glasses become accustomed to seeing the world through lenses. And I adapted to becoming progressively more deaf as I grew up, slowly building up my reper- toire of skills and strategies, especially lipreading. These were to become so ingrained that they later frustrated my attempts to listen with a cochlear implant. But being able to understand, using my tricks and strategies, became terribly precious, even as it became tremendously difficult. I was determined to behave like a hearing person. That

> I'll do anything to under- stand what someone is saying. If I have to stand on my head to lip-read someone who is standing on his head, I will.[6]
>
> – Bonnie Poitras Tucker, professor of law, who was profoundly deaf from the age of two and received an implant in adulthood

determination transformed into bluffing, into trying to pass, into hiding my deafness. It became a part of my personality, and pro- pelled me eventually toward a seemingly successful adaptation to being deaf in a hearing world.

The hearing test that I had at the age of ten was the first complete test I had. Looking at the results now, I see clues to what I could hear then. The test results showed a moderate hearing loss in both ears, starting with a 35 dB (decibel) hearing loss in the low fre- quencies. This meant that sounds had to be louder than 35 dB in those frequencies before I could hear them.[7] I may not, for exam- ple, have heard the *v* in my name. My loss in the mid frequencies sloped down to 75 dB, meaning I may not have heard a baby cry, or the *p* or *sh* sound. Then my audiogram dipped to a 100 dB loss in the high frequencies, indicating that I would not have heard whispers, or the letter *s*, or the ticking of my watch. The normal threshold levels for hearing people, who hear all these sounds, range from 0 to 25 dB. With a hearing aid boosting the volume of these sounds by as much as 60 dB, I may have heard some of them. But I still missed a lot.

After the age of ten, my hearing seems to have rapidly deteriorat- ed. I don't have a record of my audiogram from my teen years, but

I never cease to be amazed ... at how he dashes around the house "singing"; at how he understands brief messages on the telephone without any other assistance; at how he comes to find me full of excitement when he has discovered something new that he can hear (such as the gentle creaking of the refrigerator door, the sound of peeling an orange, and the chirping of a cricket).[8]

– mother of a six-year-old who has had his implant for eighteen months

I suspect that my loss moved from moderate to profound in my early teens, since I completely stopped being able to use the telephone even for short messages when I was twelve. By the time I was twenty, my audiogram showed an 85 dB loss in the low frequencies, a 100 dB loss in the mid frequencies, and a 110 dB and worse loss in the high frequencies. I would have heard no speech sounds at all (without my hearing aid) and would have seen a dog's mouth open and close but not heard his bark. I would not even have heard a phone ringing beside me. Nor would I have heard waves crashing as I walked along a beach, or leaves rustling under foot on a trail.

As a child, I had used the phone to make quick calls to my friends to arrange to meet them. These calls were actually quite rare, as I could walk everywhere in Picton and knew everyone. However, after we moved to Toronto when I was eleven, the phone became more important, while my hearing got progressively worse. Friends would call up to give me complex instructions for meeting them downtown. They would suggest that we meet at the northeast corner of Bloor and Yonge streets at two p.m. and go to the Leow's movie theater. This was quite different from "I'll meet you at the corner in fifteen minutes." There were so many possibilities for what they might say! I remember one of these calls, at the age of twelve, when I could understand nothing of what my friend was saying, even though she repeated herself over and over. I miserably handed the phone to Leah and asked her to take the message for me. I hated being dependent on others, but, even more, I hated to appear foolish. I resolved never to put myself in that kind of embarrassing situation again and stopped using the phone after that call.

When I got my cochlear implant, after being profoundly deaf for over thirty years, my hearing loss was 100 dB in the low frequencies and 120 dB and worse in the mid and high frequencies. If I was not wearing my hearing aid, I would probably hear the revving of a truck nearby, because its sound would be at about the 100 dB level, just at the point where I started to hear sounds in the low frequencies. However, a chain saw operating in front of me at the same decibel level but in the higher frequencies would be out of my range, and appear silent.

But with my hearing aid on, and my repertoire of strategies, I managed to pass as hearing and to attend regular schools, including university, and to speak. If I had been born with my profound loss, rather than progressively developing it, it is unlikely that I would have been able to do any of those things. Certainly growing up in a small town in the 1950s and 1960s, it would have been harder. But I tried to do everything that a hearing person would do, sometimes at great cost, and with mixed success.

> I am sitting in a lecture hall at York University, my heart pounding, in the grips of an anxiety attack, feeling that any moment I am going to have a heart attack. I am trapped in a room of students all listening with rapt attention to a famous professor whose writings on culture and history I loved, and who just happens to be impossible for me to lipread. He has not only a big bushy beard, but also a huge mustache. In fact his whole face seems hidden by hair. I can understand not a word he says. I want only to get out of that room fast. But I am sitting in the front row (in vain hope this would help me to hear) and cannot trust myself to slip out. Instead I sit there for the remainder of the class, with a quickly beating heart, a flush on my face, and a terror of dying.

I was the first person in my family to attend university, and my parents were pleasantly surprised and proud. I did well enough academically in high school (after a slow start) that I won a university entrance scholarship based on my grades; then I did well enough in university to maintain my scholarship. I probably got my B+ averages because I read more of the recommended texts than anyone else in my classes. I attended a liberal arts college (Glendon at York University) where most classes were, thankfully, very small so I could usually lipread the professor. Glendon was primarily a residential college, but I lived at home and went to school on the bus each day. Day students missed out on a lot, and I never made any really close friends there: I was too busy surviving. I don't remember telling anyone that I was deaf, so I didn't get any special considerations. Today, because there is more understanding and acceptance of disabilities, and because I am more open about my own hearing loss, I would probably announce to each professor that I was deaf, and I would have special notetakers assigned to me for each class. In fact, there would likely be a whole department (as there is today at the University of Toronto) with a name such as "Services to Persons with a Disability." Staff there would offer to talk to my professors to explain my hearing loss to them, and suggest ways in which they could help me to hear. They might remind them not to turn their back on the class while they were speaking – something all my professors did, with the result that there would be little holes in my understanding of their lectures marking the points at which they had turned away from me and I could not lipread them. (It was as if the sound went off and then on again.) Today, this special department would also arrange for notetakers to attend each of my classes. These notetakers would take down what the professor said and ensure that I knew when my assignments were due and when exams would be held. But, when I went to university, I managed on my own with none of these services. Sometimes I would peek at the notes of people sitting beside me in the lecture halls, and later ask to borrow them without explaining that I was deaf.

In spite of the difficulties, however, I had a large appetite for learning, and for books, and enjoyed university. I found sociology, when I took it for the first time in my freshman year, exciting, and I went on to make it my major. I loved the way it seemed to explain so much of how the world worked, of how groups and societies functioned. When I was about to graduate, I was summoned to a meeting with a favorite professor. She asked me to please consider staying on to do graduate work in the field. She felt that I had a talent for sociology. Although I was flattered, I was fatigued by university life and anxious to get into the work world.

That work world, for me, turned out to be the infant field of computers. At that time, in the late 1960s, there were no computer science university graduates, so employers were looking for people who were good at solving problems and were logical. All the strategizing and problem-solving I did as a deaf person must have been good training – I did well on the entry tests and was hired. I found programming computers great fun. It was like playing games all day long. I started working for an insurance company, where I was trained on the job, moved on to work as a consultant for the provincial government, and then joined the University of Toronto. I did tell people at work that I had a hearing impairment, so they would understand that I could not use the phone and why I might ask them to repeat things. I had no phone on my desk, and I asked secretaries to make and take calls for me when it was necessary. Other than that, I asked for and received no special accommodations. I left programming behind after a few years and moved into positions that involved analysis, project management, project planning, and research. I was repeatedly promoted by employers who appreciated the fact that I overcompensated for my deafness, often being more thorough and more hard-working than anyone else in the department.

Although the stereotype of the person who works in the computer field is of someone who sits at a computer all day and doesn't need to talk to people, this was not the case for me at all. I had to deal with meetings and project teams and conferences all the time. In one of my jobs, we had frequent peer "walk-throughs" of our work. In those "walk-throughs" (sometimes called "walk-overs" by those who were trampled by them) about a dozen of us would sit around a conference table while one of us presented our work to the

group. It might be a computer program listing, or a project propos-
al, or an analysis, or a feasibility study. The rest of the group would
ask the presenter questions and try to find flaws in the project.
When I arrived on the job and learned about this practice, I was dismayed. I was apprehensive about how I would fare. I realized I
would have to be assertive about my needs as a deaf person in order
to succeed in that environment. The first thing I asked for was that
the material being reviewed be distributed in advance, so I could
familiarize myself with it beforehand. The department agreed to this
and discovered that everyone – not just me – benefitted from being
able to review the material in advance. I also asked that people raise
their hands before they spoke so I could turn my attention to them
to lipread them, and that only one person speak at a time. I threw
myself into the practice of walk-throughs and came to love the challenge of presenting my material. Perhaps because of the contribu-
tion I was able to make, the group seemed not to mind being slowed
down by my requests for repeats and insistence that they raise their
hands and speak in turn. They often claimed that if Bev was having
trouble following, then probably others were too, but were afraid to
say so!

Unlike the term "blind" there are no legal definitions of the term
"deaf." However, total deafness, like total blindness, is rare. There is
almost always some degree of hearing ability remaining even in
those who are deaf. The three terms "hearing-impaired," "hard of
hearing," and "deaf" are often used interchangeably. Generally,
however, the first term, "hearing-impaired," embraces all those who
have a hearing loss (although those in the signing Deaf culture may
resist the label, believing they have no impairment or loss). The second term, "hard of hearing," is a gentle phrase to describe a hearing
loss and is sometimes used as a euphemism for the more blunt term
"deaf." My mother, for example, used to tell people that my father
and I were "a bit hard of hearing." However, the phrase more accurately refers to those with a hearing impairment that is mild enough
to permit them to understand speech without lipreading. Elderly

people, for example, are likely to become hard of hearing and develop some difficulty on the phone that can be helped with phone amplifiers.

The third term, "deaf," is used for those whose hearing loss is severe or profound enough that they are unable to understand speech without lipreading and unable to understand speech on the phone. Of these deaf persons, some will communicate primarily using sign language, but a larger proportion[9] will be oral deaf, like me, using lipreading to understand others, and their voices to express themselves.

Communicating by sign language rather than by speech and lipreading wasn't suggested for me until I was having trouble in the early grades at school. But by then, I was firmly established in a hearing milieu, and my speech was quite good aside from the odd mispronunciations and slurring of words. Moreover, my parents, who were mildly embarrassed about the deafness in our family, were appalled at the suggestion, made by a frustrated teacher, that I go away to a residential school for the deaf and use sign language. So I muddled along, using the little hearing I had and lipreading. Much later, when I was an adult, I did take sign language classes in night school because I was curious about the language, but I never was able to become fluent because I had no deaf friends who signed. In fact, aside from the deaf people I met during a brief period when I worked for a deaf social service agency in my thirties, I knew no other deaf people aside from those in my family and had no close deaf friends until I began to investigate a cochlear implant in my forties.

Audiologists measure the degree of hearing loss by averaging the thresholds (the softest level at which sound can be detected 50% of the time) in the frequencies of 500, 1000, and 2000 Hz, which cover the most important frequency range for understanding speech. Audiologists identify a loss as severe if the average hearing level is between 70 and 90 dB (i.e., 70 to 90 decibels above the reference point of 0 dB), and profound if the average threshold is at or above a 90 dB hearing level.[10] With a profound loss, a person would on the average hear nothing softer than 90 dB over the main frequencies of 500, 1000, and 2000 Hz. Generally, people in these two categories of hearing loss, severe and profound, where the source of the difficulty is sensorineural (i.e., in the inner ear and/or auditory nerve rather than the middle ear), are candidates for cochlear implants. If their auditory nerve itself is severed, they may be candidates for auditory brainstem implants.

Hearing loss is the most prevalent and fastest growing disability in North America, due to the aging of the population and increase in noise pollution.[11,12] Generally, one person in ten has some sort of hearing loss, and for one person in one hundred, the loss is severe or profound.[13] One in 1,000 children are born with a profound hearing loss, and one in 500 develops such a loss by the age of five.[14] In the United States, figures for the number of deaf people vary – depending on the definitions used for deafness – from approximately 2 million people who are "profoundly deaf" to 421,000 who are "deaf in both ears."[15] In Canada, statistics show that 280,000 people, or about 1% of the population, are severely or profoundly deaf.[16] Although figures are hard to obtain, estimates usually put the signing deaf at considerably less than half of the population of deaf persons. There are more oral deaf people like me than signing deaf, especially since late-deafened adults, who make up a large proportion of the deaf population, generally do not use sign language.

The majority of children with profound sensorineural deafness have a genetically caused hearing loss.[17] Even in those cases where a doctor identifies some environmental cause like an infection, scientists believe that predisposing genes play a significant role. Moreover, genetic defects may predispose adults and children to some cases of deafness caused by drugs, such as that caused by streptomycin.[18] A hereditary hearing impairment may be part of a syndrome of effects (including such traits as a premature patch of white hair), or it may appear singly without other traits. It may be recessive, meaning that it will not manifest unless both parents carry the gene, or it may be dominant, in which case it will occur at chance level (50% of the time) in the offspring of a carrier. In my own case, my genetic hearing loss was non-syndromic and was caused by a dominant gene inherited from my father.[19]

After Bob and I married, when I was twenty-two and Bob twenty-seven, we asked my ear, nose, and throat specialist about the likelihood of our children being deaf. "You can have children," he said. "If you have six children, maybe three will be deaf." I recoiled at his flippancy. Later, we visited a geneticist, who confirmed that we had a 50% chance of having a deaf child each time we conceived. Bob and I decided not to take the chance. We both saw deafness as simply too big a disability for a child to deal with, and we quickly decided to adopt. We told each other our decision was sensible and responsible, and that it was even an obvious one to make. But there was a nagging thought in my mind that I could articulate only much later (but still not answer). In not having a child of my own because he or she might be deaf, was I making a statement that a life like mine, lived without hearing, was not worth living?

I love being deaf. To me, it has been a gift. If it had not been for my deafness, I would be a different person today. And I wouldn't want to change myself for anything in the world. Because of my deafness, I've learned how to be strong, unconquerable and conscious of my self-worth in the face of extraordinary discouragement and frustration. Not only that, it's cool to be different.[20]

– Kristin Buehl, Princeton University junior who was born profoundly deaf and received an implant at the age of twenty-one

Our son, Nic, was adopted at the age of ten weeks. We were lucky, as we were able to adopt him quite soon after applying to an agency. He was an adorable healthy baby. When he was about three years old, I decided that I would like to work in the field of hearing impairment on a part-time basis. By that time, I had already had a successful career as a computer analyst and was taking time out to raise Nic. I presented myself to a service agency for deaf and hard-of-hearing people, naively expecting they would be pleased to have me work there. Instead, they were less than thrilled to have someone with a hearing impairment. They had one hard-of-hearing audiologist on staff and a few deaf people in low-paid positions; everyone else was hearing. They agreed, however, to give me a six-week course in hearing-aid technology and train me to work as a hearing-aid technician. I would fit people with hearing aids and instruct them in their use and care.

On my first day at work following the training course, I was having coffee in the staff room. I spotted the executive director of the agency and boldly marched up to him to shake his hand and introduce myself. He said, "Oh, yes, I've heard about you. I'm not sure if it's going to work."

Deflated, I said, "What do you mean?"

"The phone," he said. "You can't use the phone. That's a big problem. Our clients like to call us to talk on the phone. I don't know if it'll work out." In all my years of working in mainstream organizations, I had never encountered such an open suggestion that I could not do my job because of my hearing! I was appalled.

The director's concerns were unnecessary: I did find a way around the fact that I could not hear on the telephone. There were few calls for me, and when they did come in, a secretary was able to pass on messages for me. In most situations, clients needed to come in to see me about their problems in any case. I stayed in this job, on a part-time basis, for a couple of years, but found that it was not as satisfying as the computer field. I felt frustrated in my ability to really help my clients in the few minutes that were allocated to our appointments. So I went back to my old field, getting a job as an analyst at the University of Toronto. I am still employed there as a computing consultant and can't imagine many other more satisfying fields of work. As for the executive director – he was pushed out of his job a few years after I left. Ironically, the agency decided it was time to have a director who was deaf.

The fact that I was able to ostensibly manage in a totally auditory and oral environment in spite of my hearing loss is partly a tribute

to the complex ways in which we actually hear and understand what we hear.
There is more to hearing than what meets
the ear (as speech pathology expert
Daniel Ling says), and there is far more to
deafness than just an inability to hear.
Moreover, there was nothing exceptional
about me: there are many other oral deaf
people who have done just as well as or
better than I have with just as little or
even less hearing. Given the right combination of circumstances (that includes
when they became deaf, what sounds
they can hear, their personality, family
and other support), deaf people can
appear to manage surprisingly well in a totally oral and auditory
environment. Some can even pass as hearing, the way I did.

> Although I do not think
> about it much, I do take
> pride in the fact that I
> communicate orally. It's
> unquestionably an
> achievement to be able to
> communicate with hearing
> people on something
> close to their own
> terms.[21]
>
> – *Lew Golan, who*
> *became profoundly deaf*
> *from meningitis at the*
> *age of six and received*
> *an implant fifty-five*
> *years later*

Many of the tricks I used to communicate in spite of my hearing
loss are also tricks that I and others use to manage with the necessarily limited information given by cochlear implants. My collection
of strategies included lipreading, as well as the information provided by contextual cues, rules of articulation, and vibrations. The most
important of these was lipreading or, as it is sometimes called,
"speechreading," because it involves more than the lips. If people
wore sunglasses, for example, I would have trouble understanding
what they said, as I needed to see the expressions in their eyes while
they were talking. I would startle them by saying, "Please take off
your sunglasses. I can't hear you." I became adept at speechreading
(unless the person had hair covering his mouth, like my history professor, or had a heavy accent, or mumbled, or spoke through gritted
teeth or with a pipe in his mouth). I learned it "on the job" from
early childhood. Not all deaf children can develop good
speechreading skills, however. One study of hearing-impaired ten-
year-olds showed that their ability to lipread was significantly cor-
related with their visual memory for complex shapes.[22] A man I

know, who was born with a moderate to severe hearing loss and now uses sign language as his main mode of communication, sadly recalls being berated as a child for his poor lipreading ability. We do not completely understand why some people seem to have a talent for it, and others just don't. We do know, however, that those who are deafened in adulthood generally have a much harder time learning to speechread than those who learn the trick from childhood.[23]

Not surprisingly, lipreading skill is one prognosticator for relatively successful use of a cochlear implant.[24] Those who can do well with limited sound information, using whatever tools they can, will more likely do well with their cochlear implant. The attributes of a successful speechreader are similar to those of a successful cochlear implant user: flexible and alert, yet relaxed. Ann Perry and Richard Silverman are really describing a successful implant wearer, too, when they say, "The secret of successful speechreading lies in the ability to grasp an idea intuitively and develop its meaning without attempting to follow every word."[25] When I was learning to hear with my implant, my adaptations to deafness stood me in good stead, at the same time that they frustrated my attempts to just listen.

Spoken English contains forty phonemes (or sounds from which words are formed), only about one-third of which are clearly visible on the face of a speaker.[26,27] Languages other than English may be easier or harder to understand by speechreading. For example, tonal languages such as Mandarin Chinese may be difficult to lipread because tonal variations in words are used to convey meaning. In the English language, many words look identical on the lips, and it is easy for people to confuse words and misconstrue a whole sentence if they are relying solely on speechreading.

The deaf author Henry Kisor called his autobiography *What's That Pig Outdoors?* in honor of a gross error in lipreading that he once made. His five-year-old son had asked him, "What's that big loud noise?" and Henry obligingly went to the window to look for that pig outdoors. If you repeat the child's question in front of a mirror, it's easy to see how Henry made this mistake.

If only one-third of phonemes are clearly readable on the face, how can I and other oral deaf people manage to understand more than one-third of what people say? The answer is that in addition to information from reading the face of the speaker, I can use two other tools: contextual cues, and the rules for how words sound.

I can achieve closure (filling in the blanks, adding two plus two to make five) by using contextual information. English is a highly redundant language, and using this redundancy, I can resolve ambiguities in speech by understanding its context, waiting and listening to the rest of a sentence, or perhaps the next sentence. Just as a hearing person figures out whether a word was "to" or "too" from its context in a sentence, so I will figure out if a word is "bat" or "bad" (both of which look the same on the lips) from how it is used in a sentence or set of sentences. That is why most people, if they have enough hearing to understand 50% of single-syllable words in a test, can generally understand 100% of the sentences in a test.[28] None of us, whether hearing or hearing-impaired, really need to understand every word in a sentence to make sense of it, as long as we have some language proficiency.

There is only a small jump from using context to achieve closure, however, and bluffing. Sometimes (much less frequently since I got my implant), I will guess at what someone is saying, with embarrassing results. I will add two and two to come up not with five, but with ten. Other times, I will make a split-second decision that what I didn't understand was not important enough to ask for a repetition. In those cases, I may simply coast and possibly pretend that I have understood when I have not.

There are rules for how words sound in a certain language, or rules of language articulation that I have absorbed unconsciously, and I can quickly call them up on the fly to resolve ambiguities. So, for example, in English, the *a* vowel is shorter in duration when it comes before the consonant *t* than when it comes before the consonant *d*. This kind of timing clue can be very useful, not only in the case of speechreading, but also in the case of hearing with my cochlear implant, where timing-based sound information can be relatively easy to grasp. Similarly, the rhythm of speech can be important. The sentence, "How are you?" for example, has a certain rhythm to it, a rise and fall in pitch and a change in speech duration that helps me to recognize the question and respond correctly, even if I have not understood every word. When I was little, however, I often answered the question "How old are you?" by saying, "I'm fine, thanks."

Robert Shannon, of the House Ear Institute in Los Angeles, uses a fuzzy picture of Abraham Lincoln to demonstrate that we do not need to understand everything to comprehend the gist of what is being said. Dr. Shannon shows his audience a picture of a cultural icon, Abraham Lincoln. It is a very coarse grainy version of the portrait on the U.S. five-dollar bill, "pixelated" (returned to its basic digital picture elements or pixels) so that it is really just a collection of black and gray squares. Yet even with a very vague, partial picture of Lincoln, the audience is able to draw on their visual memories to fill in the blanks, and say, "I know that's Abraham Lincoln." The full picture has been presented to them so many times in their past that it has become part of their visual memory. So too can those of us with a hearing impairment somehow draw on our auditory memory (if any exists) to fill in the blanks and understand speech and other sounds based on what we have heard in the past. Auditory memory is especially important for successful use of a cochlear implant (where the signal is partial and "pixelated" too), and it may be weak in those who like me have been profoundly deaf for a long time.

It helps deaf people to have good language proficiency in general in order to put the information they obtain from speechreading together with the information they derive from context and rules of articulation. Fortunately for me, I was able to ameliorate the effects of deafness by being an avid reader from an early age. As a result, my language skills were good. These skills, combined with the inexperience of most people with deafness, made it easier for me to pass as hearing. Most people outside my immediate family did not understand how little I actually heard, nor did they understand the restrictions my poor hearing necessarily placed upon me.

When I was about thirteen years old, I found a poor couple who were so desperate for a babysitter that they took me on. I think I answered an ad posted on a grocery store bulletin board. I have a vague recollection of my mother making the call for me and explaining to the parents that I was a "bit hard of hearing." They apparently said that was no problem and asked me to come to babysit their children the following Saturday night. I was hired. I was elated. I was looking forward to all the money I was going to earn for makeup and clothes. When the Saturday rolled around, I made my way to the strange neighborhood of their low-rise apartment. Their place was plain but warm, and their greetings were effusive. They showed me the plate of cookies, and the bowl of potato chips, and the fridge, and said those magic words: "Make yourself at home." They were dressed up glamorously, he in a dark suit, and she in a low-cut evening dress. She came out of the bedroom, smelling of heavy perfume, to ask him to zip up the back of her dress. I felt privy to something sexual, something exciting.

Before they left, I told them casually that I did not hear very well, and that I did not use the phone. They just nodded and smiled, and said not to worry about it. They must have thought I meant that I would not use the phone to call my friends all evening. Or maybe they just thought I was being shy (hence their encouraging smiles and admonishments not to worry). In fact, they were clueless.

I felt wonderfully free when they finally backed out the door and were gone. I was alone. In an apartment filled with books. And food. All to myself. I started munching on the chips, helped myself to some pop in the fridge, and got down on the floor to start an examination of their book cases. After flipping through some of their books (nothing about sex, unfortunately), I made a quick check of the children sleeping peacefully in their bedrooms, then settled in front of the television set. About an hour later, I was happily engrossed in a movie on television when they came rushing in the door. The parents had come back already! Moreover, they were very upset. The mother rushed to the children's bedroom and came back out cradling her youngest in her arms to confront me angrily. The father was furious. I was bewildered. He said to me accusingly, "We phoned, and phoned, and phoned. Why didn't you answer?" I said, "I don't hear well. I can't use the phone." He took a few seconds to absorb this, then just nodded with annoyance and took out his wallet. He thrust some money at me, and then I picked myself up from my comfortable place on the couch, and left the potato chips and books and freedom behind. That was my first and last babysitting job.

One method of quickly giving a deaf child language proficiency is called Cued Speech. This is a system that uses a hand movement to the face to help distinguish between sounds that look alike on the lips. For example, to distinguish between the words "bat" and "bad," I would (if I cued) speak the former with five fingers raised to my chin to signify the *t*, whereas I would speak the latter with one finger to my chin to signify the *d*. Because the system of cueing consists of only eight handshapes in four different locations near the face, the system itself can be learned in a matter of weeks. Both children and adults with hearing impairments can use Cued Speech, although I never did. It has many proponents in North America and was developed by Dr. R. Orin Cornett at Gallaudet (an American liberal arts college for the deaf) in the 1960s. It is, however, less commonly used in Canada than in some other countries such as Australia and France. [29]

As my experiment with tapping a knife against a wine glass showed after I got my cochlear implant, sensing vibrations, in addition to speechreading, and using contextual cues and rules of language articulation was yet another way in which there was more to my hearing than what met my ear. I could feel the thud of the knife against the glass and feel the glass vibrate rapidly to indicate a high-pitched sound. Some deaf people enjoy loud music by holding their hands on a balloon while music is playing, and many enjoy dancing to loud music that they can feel in their bodies. In the case of very loud sounds, just as the hairs in the normal inner ear bend in response to sound, so too may the hairs on my skin bend slightly in response, and alert me.

When I read the newspaper at breakfast with my implant turned off, if my dog, Blossom, barks to tell me that someone is at the door, I hear her not with my ears, but by sensing the vibrations in the newspaper I am holding. After he became deaf, Beethoven used to place a wooden stick between his teeth and rest the other end on his piano in order to hear music through vibrations. Similarly, the deaf American inventor Thomas Alva Edison, who perfected the phonograph, bit on his phonograph's wooden frame to pick up the sound of music playing.[30] Edison was also an accomplished telegrapher, detecting the sounds of a telegraph machine through his sense of touch.[31]

Vibrotactile aids for the deaf make use of this similarity of hearing to touch and our ability to receive sound information through vibrations. These aids are electronic devices that consist of a small vibrator strapped to a deaf person's chest or arm or hand, and a processor and microphone. The microphone picks up sounds, and the processor sorts and converts them into appropriate electrical impulses that go to the vibrator to stimulate (or tickle) the skin. There are also electrotactile aids that work similarly, but they use electrodes rather than vibrators to stimulate the skin. For some children and adults who are severely to profoundly deaf and cannot use a cochlear implant, tactile aids can supplement speechreading and help in developing intelligible speech.[32]

Evelyn Glennie provides a remarkable demonstration of how well vibrations can convey sound information. Glennie

> If I had a deaf child I would teach him by holding him against my body all the time, so he could feel the vibrations of my speech. I would lie with his hands on my throat, hold him against my heart, lay him on the piano so he could learn about sound and music from the air. With a hearing child, I'd do the same. Your ears are just one of a multitude of ways of experiencing sound.[33]
>
> *– Evelyn Glennie, deaf Scottish percussionist, who does not want (nor appear to need) a "cure" for her deafness*

is a deaf Scottish percussionist who has developed an incredible means of hearing and performing her music in spite of her profound deafness. She feels the vibrations emanating from her music. Perhaps it is because of rather than in spite of her profound hearing loss that she has developed such remarkable talent. Glennie says in her autobiography, *Good Vibrations*, that she has never wanted a cure for her deafness: "I had learnt to cope with my silent world, and felt that my own ways of listening to music gave me a sensitivity that I far preferred to the 'normal' way of hearing that I had experienced as a tiny child . ... I didn't want to lose that special gift."[34] When I saw her perform at Roy Thomson Hall in Toronto, her feet were shoeless, so she could better feel the vibrations of the orchestra around her and of her own music making. Stroking and smashing bells, xylophones, and drums, she appeared to be in a trance. When she moved, it was with awesome energy and passion; her performance was electrifying to watch.

Before I got my cochlear implant, I found the very loud rock music that my teenage son played unbearable. I would feel it throbbing throughout my body. I would want him to turn it down (or even better, shut it off) immediately! Now that I have more hearing with a cochlear implant, this loud pounding music does not bother me nearly as much. I puzzled over this, because the music is much louder to me with my implant. Then I realized that in the past, I had found the loud music threatening. With almost no hearing, I had felt the music more than I had heard it. And the vibrations reminded me of the way my family called my father when they wanted his attention: by stamping their feet so he could feel the vibrations. I was highly sensitive to these rock music beats because I realized they could be a signal or even a warning that I was in danger.

Adult cochlear implant users frequently observe that their new hearing makes them feel "alive." The reason for this also helps to explain what it feels like to be deaf. It hints at how terribly stressful deafness can be emotionally and physically in spite of our ability to call on all the tricks of speechreading, contextual information, rules of language articulation, and vibrations.

As Donald Ramsdell describes it in *Hearing and Deafness*,[35] there is a primitive level on which our hearing operates to connect each of us to our surroundings. Even if we are not consciously aware of the sounds in our environment, on a basic level, these sounds tell us we are in a world that is alive around us. We are unconsciously aware of people moving about us, of noises outside our window, of machinery working. This level of hearing also helps us to stay in a state of readiness to react to sounds that may signify danger or that require some action on our part. When that connection is cut off, we may feel the deadness many deafened people describe as coming over them. Our environment has become dead, and we may also feel to some extent that we too have become dead. With my implant turned off, I feel like I am soundlessly walking down stairs and passing through rooms like a ghost. Ramsdell, studying soldiers deafened in the Second World War, found that they repeatedly complained that the world seemed dead.[36]

Virtually all people who receive cochlear implants obtain hearing on this primitive level and can appreciate a greater connectedness with their environment and a greater sense of security and peace. That is why even the earliest crude single-channel implants gave such tremendous joy to their wearers. In my own case, although I heard environmental sounds with my hearing aid, they were muted, and I didn't hear them all. When I threw a stone into a stream, I might not hear it splash. Now, I often walk downstairs in the morning with my processor not yet turned on because the world still comes on too loud, and I need to ease into the day. My footsteps make no sound hitting the stairs; it is as if I am without substance, floating, and airy, as if I would leave no footprints in the sand on a beach were I to turn around and look. The greater sense of connectedness and security I feel with my implant turned on is one of the reasons why, after the first few days, I took such a deep pleasure in my hearing with it, at the same time as I sometimes felt disappointed that I could not understand more of what I heard.

> I was so conscious of my surroundings [before getting my implant] that my concentration level was always set on high. If I wasn't paying attention, I could have been hit by a truck – and never heard it coming. My metabolism was in super warp speed ... I was hyperactive, high-strung, and ... thin![37]
>
> – Joanne Syrja, with tongue firmly in cheek

Before I got my cochlear implant, I needed to be constantly on the alert for things that would require my attention: people approaching me from behind, people starting up a conversation with me, ambulances racing through the street. The list is endless. Being on the alert meant picking up subtle cues in my environment, such as a slight movement of air from a door opening, vibrations in the floor under my feet from a person approaching me, cars slowing down and moving to the side of the road for an oncoming ambulance, small changes in the mood of a group of people indicating that an announcement is being made, people looking at me questioningly when someone else has spoken to me. I felt much less of a need to be constantly on the alert for these sorts of clues once I had more hearing with a cochlear implant. Hearing made life a little more easeful.

It can be emotionally devastating to be unable to understand what people are saying. It is lonely to be in a crowd and not understand what's going on, not understand why people have grown somber or have burst into laughter. This inability to understand others can be frustrating and demeaning.

> I am in an eighth grade geography class, at the age of twelve. The teacher has called on me to answer a question about the whereabouts of some place on the crinkly map she has rolled down over the blackboard. I do not understand the name of the place she wants me to locate (proper names have always been hard to understand because they have no contextual clues that I can grab), so I say, "I don't know where it is." She has no inkling that I am deaf. I hadn't told her, and she hadn't noticed the office record indicating my hearing impairment.

She is stern and annoyed, and asks me to come up to the map and locate something else. I am flustered and do not understand the name of that place either. I am aware that the kids around me are making a lot of noise. She tells them to be quiet and let me figure it out myself (as if I could have understood their called-out answers). She will not let me sit down and continues repeating the question a second and a third time. Then she gives up on me and, pointing at the map with her wooden pointer, says disgustedly, "Don't you even know where the equator is?" I feel mortified.

Anger, depression, withdrawal, and isolation are common responses to hearing loss, for those deafened in adulthood. Moreover, the literature on the subject shows that adults with hearing impairments are likely to be more maladjusted emotionally than are hearing people.[38] We may believe that others are talking about us when we do not understand their voices, and we may make wild guesses about what we think they have said. As the British psychiatrist Anthony Storr says, "People who become profoundly deaf often seem to be even more cut off from others than those who are blind. Certainly they are more likely to become suspicious of their nearest and dearest. Deafness, more than blindness, is apt to provoke paranoid delusions of being disparaged, deceived, and cheated."[39]

Denial is another common emotional response to hearing loss. The average length of time between the suspicion of a hearing loss and an audiological assessment is five years for adults[41] and 11.5 months for children.[42] Part of this delay may be due to other factors, such as the casual (or even ill-informed) treatment of a hearing loss by a family doctor, but

Our reaction to hearing about his deafness was relief. We'd spent so many inconclusive months worrying about what was wrong with him, so many visits to the pediatrician being accused of hysteria, that learning that he was deaf sort of enabled us to "start".[40]

– Celeste Coleon, France, mother of three-year-old Max, who was diagnosed as deaf at around eighteen months and received an implant a year later

there may also be a tendency to deny a hearing loss, or to blame it on other causes (for example, people mumble too much or a child is simply inattentive, or a mother is a worrier).[43]

Today, there is still some stigma attached to deafness, and this stigma can encourage the denial of deafness. We have only to read the hearing-aid advertisements that crow about devices so small as to be invisible to others to witness the social attitude that says deafness is something to be ashamed of and hidden. And there are the advertisements (more common in the past) for hearing-aid salesmen who will fit you with a hearing aid "in the privacy of your own home." The rise of Deaf pride in North America began on the campus of Gallaudet University in 1988 following the humiliating statement by the chairperson of the university's board of trustees that "deaf people are not ready to function in a hearing world." This pride has challenged the notion that deafness is shameful. Like the gay liberation movement, the women's movement, and Black pride, the Deaf pride movement has empowered people who have long been discriminated against. Along with all others with a hearing impairment, I am a beneficiary of the Deaf pride movement.

I seemed to manage with my profound hearing loss and developed a good repertoire of tricks and strategies. When I was a teenager, a close friend, in a burst of late-night honesty, confessed that when she first met me, I seemed to put up a wall around myself, and that I appeared to keep people at a distance so they could not get to know me well. Now, looking back on her observation, I believe it was the tricks and strategies that were the bricks and mortar of my fortress. I could not let people come close enough to see that beyond the tricks and strategizing was a very deaf person.

There were consequences, however, for trying to live as a hearing person with a profound level of deafness. As I got older, I found it harder to pay those consequences. I was exhausted at the end of a day at work filled with stressful meetings and speechreading. I was on edge trying to be alert to all the movements and sounds around me so as not to be taken by surprise. My social life was constricted by the difficulty I had following the free flow of conversations in groups. I avoided concerts and parties.

My deafness was also increasingly restricting the social life of Bob. He's gregarious, with passions that include singing and folk music. I was too dependent on him to do what my mother had done for my father: make phone calls for me and take my messages, and explain what I missed in conversations. Moreover, the guilty feelings of my mother at having a deaf child had become transformed in Bob into guilt for taking pleasure from music and social gatherings when I was left out. Unfortunately, the hearing, as the deaf poet David Wright says, absorb a large part of the impact of deafness in a family. Too often, I felt a seething anger about my deafness (which was sometimes projected onto other matters and other people), and a suspicion of those around me (because of what I wrongly thought I heard). There is no doubt that by the time I was in my forties, I was ready for any improvement I could get in my hearing. Even an ability to better hear environmental sounds and lipread with more ease would be wonderful. I needed to cut myself (and my family) some slack.

> I am watching two of my women friends at a party. In a room of thirty people, they are the only deaf people aside from myself. They had lost their hearing in adulthood and have not been deaf for as long as I have. They are staying together, talking animatedly to each other, using some sign language to ease the communication flow. Then, as often happens at parties at my house, because of Bob's love of music, with encouragement from him, people break out into song. The deaf women, after a few minutes, take note of the singing, look confused for a moment, then smile at each other and at those around them, and resume their animated talking and gesturing. I watch them, feeling sad. Although they are together, they are also apart from the group. I feel a sadness on their behalf for being in the midst of such warm, beautiful music, and seeming to be

oblivious to it. This is what it is like to be deaf for me: to be different, and unreceptive in the midst of talk, of song, of noise, and other audible expressions of the soul. This for me is the essence of deafness: being lonely in a crowd.

DEAFNESS IN THE FAMILY

About deafness, I know everything and nothing.
Everything, if forty years' first-hand experience is to
count. Nothing, when I realize how little I have had
to do with the converse aspects of deafness – the
other half of the dialogue. Of that side my wife
knows more than I.[1]
– David Wright

Deafness has profoundly affected my original family, as well as the family I have created with my husband and son. It has made Bob feel guilty and resentful at times; it has made me feel dependent, and I have resented that dependence. I think deafness has also fostered personality traits in me that sometimes complicate relationships within my family.

My deafness and that of my father had a big impact on my older sister, Leah, when she was growing up, and I think it helped to shape her personality. She grew into the role of a kind-hearted "helper," for both my father and me. Lou Ann Walker, the hearing child of deaf parents and the author of the wonderful autobiography, *A Loss for Words*, reminds me of Leah. Like Lou Ann Walker, Leah has a tendency to rescue people and put others' needs ahead of her own. I think this has something to do with the position she was placed in in our family. She sometimes stood in for my mother, even making business phone calls for my father when she was a child. Later she would make phone calls for me, too, and became privy to some of my complex social arrangements and teenage intrigues. And, as my older sister, she was often charged with looking after me (and looking out for me). She sometimes resented that – and having to share a bedroom with me! I know my deafness affected her greatly when we were growing up, and that she is now moved by my ability to hear more. I know too, from what she has told me, that she felt deeply guilty at being spared from deafness while I was not.

And mine was not the only deafness in the family. When Leah was about five (two years before I was born), my father accidentally slammed a heavy door on her baby finger. That would have been bad enough, but when she screamed in pain, he didn't hear her and walked away. It was my mother who heard her and came running to open the door and free her finger.

I have my own story about being affected by my father's deafness. I remember when I was about five or six, climbing into my father's truck and going for a ride with him and his driver to a gravel quarry on the outskirts of town. I loved to go places with my father in his fire-engine-red truck. It was an adventure to ride high up in the cab of the truck, sitting on the lumpy seat between him and his driver. Once at the quarry, I went off to explore and play in the gravel and sand, while my father and the driver did their business. After a while, I tired of playing in the hot shadeless yard and looked for them. I called out but couldn't find them. I remember feeling that it was no use calling out, because my father wouldn't hear me. What I didn't realize was that because of my own poor hearing, I may not have heard my father or the driver call me either. I gave up and set off for home. I remember trudging the mile or two beside the highway, feeling dejected and betrayed. At home, my father was waiting for me, and my mother was furious at him for having left me. I still don't know the full story behind that unforgettable day, but I date from it my loss of faith in my father and his ability to protect me.

I had an uneasy relationship with my father when I was growing up. I was repelled by his deafness, which was more severe than mine until I reached late adolescence. I saw in him and his apparent weakness and dependence on others my own future. It frightened me. I still shudder when I remember how we stamped our feet on the floor to get his attention. I found it demeaning; even now, I don't know why. My father and I did not discuss our shared disability, and I don't know how he felt about my deafness. I was closer to my hearing mother and knew more about her feelings, both the guilt she felt and the protectiveness.

My mother's feeling of guilt is a common reaction of parents on learning their child is deaf. Parents may feel there was something they did to cause their child's deafness. Or they might refuse to believe it is permanent. They may also feel especially obliged to protect their child from further harm. David Luterman[2] tells the heart-wrenching story of one mother who each morning would wake up convinced her child could now hear, run into the child's bedroom, and try to wake her by calling out to her. When the child did not respond, the mother would feel devastated all over again. This mother badly needed support from others in helping her to come to terms with her child's deafness.

Bob likes to draw a parallel between his own situation and that of the spouse of someone in a wheelchair. "When people see a married woman in a wheelchair, with her husband behind her," he says, "they know her husband will have a lot to deal with because of her disability. They probably will feel compassion for him. But when they see a deaf woman with a hearing husband, they just don't understand the problems he faces." I think he's right. He and other partners of deaf people, as well as other hearing family members, often feel unappreciated, and their problems go unrecognized. Moreover, we both think the problems of living with someone deaf are more pervasive than those of someone living with a partner in a wheelchair. Deafness affects our ability to communicate, and communication is at the heart of family life.

Deafness can put a crushing burden on a marriage between a hearing and a deaf person and cause it to fail.[3] Bonnie Tucker told in her autobiography, *The Feel of Silence*, of how her husband decided after seventeen years of marriage that he no longer wanted to be married to a deaf woman. He found the inconvenience and limitations unbearable. In fact, he once stopped speaking to her for several weeks, because he was fed up with having to come to find her rather than being able to call out her name from another room. When she asked him later if he would have left a partner who had become paraplegic as a result of an accident, he unflinchingly answered that he would. He said the disability would be his partner's, not his, and he shouldn't need to live with it.

Tucker claims to know of very few successful marriages between deaf women and hearing men. However, she knows of many good marriages between deaf men and hearing women. I suspect that men, because of their socialization, may have difficulty assuming the nurturing role demanded of a hearing husband to a deaf woman, whereas women may find that role a bit easier. I have been fortunate in that nurturing has come more easily to Bob than it does to many men. He was an elementary school teacher and is now a teacher of English as a Second Language to adults. A caring teacher, he teaches his adult students (immigrants to Canada) more than just English: he also listens to their personal problems and helps them negotiate government bureaucracies. Nonetheless, my deafness has sometimes caused a terrible strain on him that he has found difficult to bear. In some ways, the burden of my deafness is harder for him to bear than for me, because I have become acclimatized to it since childhood, whereas he has not.

I try to put myself in Bob's shoes. I close my eyes and imagine myself married to someone with a major disability. Someone in a wheelchair, for example. Someone who has grown up using a wheelchair and has a thousand tricks for dealing with it, even though he sometimes comes to unpassable steps (literally and figuratively) and gets frustrated and angry. I don't know how to handle being married to this person. I don't know how to help him or even when to help him. I feel I am bound by his wheelchair too, but I don't know where to get the kind of support that he is getting from others in his situation. I don't have the adaptations he has, and I feel myself lost and out of control. I feel helpless yet wanting to help. I feel needy myself, yet obligated to respond to his needs. That must be the way Bob feels. And I think: being married to someone deaf is worse.

Some time after I received my cochlear implant, I learned that Bob was telling people how much it had changed his life. He told them how much easier his life was, how pleased he was that he no longer needed to spend his lunch hour making phone calls on my behalf, how he felt more comfortable in social gatherings knowing that I could follow without his help. He told them how he felt freer, even liberated.

Bob's sense of freedom and relief that I am now hearing more highlights the problems that he experienced in living with me before I got my implant. We were fortunate in that my deafness did not come as a surprise during our marriage – I was deaf when we met. In many marriages between a deaf person and a hearing person, the deafness comes later, as a surprise, a pail of cold water, and the marriage flounders and dies. I know of many such marriages. Although Bob put up with making dates with me over the phone through my mother before we married, and knew he was marrying a deaf woman, he did not, however, fully realize how much his life would be affected by my deafness.

Bob was sometimes constrained in doing the things he enjoys – and felt guilty when he did enjoy them. He would feel trapped between the guilt at going to a music concert or a social event with

> A significant change has developed in our casual conversation. There is more "small talk" and "asides" – communication that gives humor and color to the day. ... In the usual friction of daily living it provides a subtle lubricant.[4]
>
> *– Frank Martin on the changes resulting from his wife Joyce's hearing with a cochlear implant*

me – knowing that I was not enjoying myself – and the resentment at passing up the event and staying home. If it were a clear-cut case of my not wanting to attend the event, it would be easier for him. But so often my position was ambivalent, mirroring my ambivalence as a deaf person in a hearing milieu. I would want to go, but fear I would feel cheated because I would not hear well enough to enjoy the event. And because he is a kind and sensitive man, Bob would feel guilty about his resentment.

In social situations, I was sometimes lost, unable to follow a quick change of speaker. Sometimes people would direct their conversation to Bob alone, thinking I would not understand. I would usually say nothing, but it was hurtful to be ignored in this way. Bob would often good-naturedly take it on himself to repeat the other person's conversation to me if he realized I was not following. Then sometimes my resentment would spill over onto him. Pauline Ashley, the wife of Lord Jack Ashley, who became totally deaf while a member of the British Parliament, tells of people talking directly to her when their message was meant for her husband. She says that when this happened, she would pointedly look at her husband while the speaker was talking, to encourage the speaker to do the same.[5] It often worked. When I became friends with some deaf people and attended social functions with them, I was dismayed to find that I too fell into the easy habit of directing my speech to a hearing spouse (knowing that I would be understood) rather than to his or her deaf partner (who might not understand). I would – I hope – usually catch myself.

Social gatherings would sometimes leave me feeling frustrated, and later, after everyone had left or while we were driving home, I might ask Bob to repeat to me what different people had said. I would want to hear all the details. This, of course, put a strain on Bob and on our relationship. We slowly cut back on the number of these social occasions, sometimes finding excuses for not attending.

Once when we were having problems in the family, we had family therapy, but with very limited success. I remember at our first meeting, an eminent psychiatrist explaining something to us in a soft voice, and when I told him I was deaf and did not understand him, he turned to Bob and said, "You explain it to her." We were so intimidated by him, and so needy, that neither of us was able to tell him I required him to talk directly to me. We continued to visit him for several months, and he continued to be insensitive about my hearing loss.

I have developed some personality traits in response to deafness that have made me admittedly difficult to live with at times – or if I haven't developed them solely because of my deafness, they have at least been nourished by it. I am a perfectionist. I need to be in control and to map things out in advance to forestall surprises. I would like to say that I am like a blind person who needs to get the lay of the land, but I've met a lot of very relaxed blind people who have dashed that analogy! Unable to hear perfectly, I tried to make all else around me perfect; afraid of missing things I didn't hear, I developed keen powers of concentration and intensity. While making it easier for me to successfully cope with my deafness, these traits have also made it difficult for others who share my life. The deaf poet David Wright says that like the prospect of hanging, a disability concentrates the facilities wonderfully.[6] The down-side of that is that for the spouse especially, it may feel like the hanging is about to begin at any moment!

Before I got my implant, the telephone was a big problem for both me and my family. I couldn't use it, and I relied on Bob and our son, Nic, to help me with it. That meant that Bob needed to help me make social arrangements if I wanted to go out with friends; he needed to make my medical appointments, make all the calls to service people to get appliances fixed, and do many of the other things that had to be transacted over the phone. Nic would be unable to call to tell me that he would be late for dinner or needed to be picked up – although he would sometimes phone a neighbor and ask her to give me the message.

I resented my dependence on Bob for help with the telephone, and he resented needing to help me, although he was usually gracious

I am not saying life is perfect. ... Harvey often complains, for example, about half-hour phone conversations I have that are then relayed to him in only a few sentences. Large gatherings are still a problem. Harvey says that in a large group we sometimes forget that he exists. This may seem true, but I am a hearing person, and if someone with normal hearing goes on talking I can't stop them![7]

– *Jos Patel, whose husband, Harvey, hears with a cochlear implant*

about it. When he talked on the phone to our friends or my sister, Leah, or other family members, I would badger him after he hung up, hungry for details of the conversation. He would prefer to give me a very brief summary of what was said, but, I have to admit that often this was not enough for me.

Other couples have worked out arrangements to allow the deaf partner to use the phone. For example, some deaf people pick up the receiver and ask their hearing partner to listen nearby on an extension phone (or extra receiver). The hearing person then mouths the speaker's words to the deaf partner who responds as if he or she heard the conversation over the phone. I tried that system a couple of times but felt it was too great an imposition on Bob. I did, however, use a relay system provided by the local telephone company. This service provided operators who would relay spoken messages from people talking on regular phones back to me on my TTY (a small device with a keyboard and a screen that allows a deaf or non-speaking person to transmit messages across the telephone lines). The relay system was helpful to me and reduced my dependence on Bob. But I was still dependent on someone else, only now it was an operator! It rankled, and I often resented the slowness of the operators' typing or their obvious errors in transmitting what was said. My skill on the telephone now with my cochlear implant is one that I am fiercely proud of, because it gives me a sense of independence the lack of which used to grate on me terribly.

After we were accepted by our local adoption agency, we needed to satisfy the agency's social worker that my deafness would not prevent me from hearing a baby cry. When the word came that we could bring Nic home in a few days, we excitedly ran out and bought not just a crib and red sleepers and an old-fashioned baby carriage, but also a special device that picked up and greatly amplified any sounds he made in his bedroom. When he was safely installed in his new crib, I could hear his cries, and his sneezes and giggles too, if I turned the speaker up loud enough. I could hear him from any room in the house, and I suspect the neighbors heard him too!

Even from toddlerhood, Nic understood that I could not hear well and helped me out, sweetly explaining to people that "mommy's ears don't work" when I seemed to miss conversational cues and was unaware of it. Later, he uncomplainingly made phone calls and took messages for me, although when he hit his teens, some of my messages went astray. I tried not to ask him to make or take too many of my calls. I was concerned about treating him, as someone once put it, as a portable assistive listening device. Some children who are used heavily in this way by their deaf parents come to resent it when they are grown. So far, thankfully, Nic has shown none of this resentment.

Our beloved Nic had a relatively untroubled, easy childhood and was in many ways a model child: outgoing, kind-hearted, and athletic. He has brought Bob and me much joy. When he hit adolescence, my deafness became more obviously a problem for him. His adoption also weighed heavily on his mind. Adoption and deafness were volatile ingredients to add to the usual stew of adolescent stresses.

When Nic grew into his teens, I think he was embarrassed by my voice, especially if I called him loudly and screeched. He seemed embarrassed that I was different and he became less accommodating. He used that major tool of adolescent rebellion – hair – as a weapon against me. He grew his dark brown bangs so long that they covered his face and mouth, and I had trouble understanding his explanations for why he was late for dinner, or had skipped school, or lost his notebook. I was relieved when he began to tie his long hair back in a sleek ponytail.

Nic was not very enthusiastic about my getting a cochlear implant, especially after he met some cochlear implant users and thought they were not managing much better than I was with my hearing aid. I could understand that. After all, he had never known me as other than his deaf mother, and neither of us fully understands even today the impact of my deafness on him. This was my natural state for him. He was also afraid that something would go wrong during the surgery.

> I was somewhat surprised when I heard my son's voice for the first time through my implant – it sounded unfamiliar because he had grown from a small child to a "real" boy in the intervening years when my hearing changed so markedly, and I had never heard his more mature voice.[9]
>
> – *cochlear implant user Donna Sorkin*

Pauline Ashley says that her husband's deafness "worried" their two older daughters, but that their youngest daughter, who was eighteen months old when her father went deaf, took it in stride.[8] Ashley says her youngest daughter simply told her friends how best to speak to her father, and they just as simply accepted her instructions.

It was often easier for Nic to talk to Bob than to me when it was something he was embarrassed about, or something he wanted to talk about quietly and get it over with. This could be a problem if it happened too often: I would feel left out and resentful, especially if the discussion took place right in front of me and I couldn't follow it. But I tried (usually) to see it from Nic's point of view, and understand that he had his own needs, too, and could not always be thinking of how to accommodate mine.

Before I received my cochlear implant, conversation around the dinner table was becoming more and more difficult. Perhaps it was because I was getting older and finding it harder to be as quick in my lipreading as I used to be, or perhaps it was because of the nature of the conversations. If they were the typical defensive, adolescent discussions about school and friends, Bob and Nic sometimes couldn't seem to slow down enough for me. I felt angry that I was being left out of important family discussions and decisions. One researcher observes that any hearing-impaired adult living with two or more hearing adults will experience a social handicap because there will be conversations from which he or she will inevitably be excluded[10] – and this was certainly becoming true in our family.

It was Bob, early in our marriage, who had encouraged me to be more open about my deafness. It seemed like common sense to him, that I should explain my disability to others, rather than have them believe me to be rude or foolish. He didn't feel the stigma and shame that I felt about deafness; he had not grown up trying to pass as hearing. He was less affected by old social attitudes that encouraged people to view disabilities with embarrassment and even revulsion. Over the years, he helped me face the fact that bluffing and passing were not serving me well. It was a slow but steady progression that I made with his help. It started with my simply telling people about my hearing loss, then asking for the accommodations I needed: "Please don't cover your mouth. Can we turn the lights up? Can we rearrange the seating?" My progress culminated in my obtaining a cochlear implant with his encouragement, and recognizing how much I needed it.

I did wonder, however, when I was considering a cochlear implant, if my dependency on Bob was something that had attracted him to me when we married, and if there would be a problem with our relationship if I became less needy. I wondered if some delicate balance of needs and strengths might be disrupted. Looking at what the experts have to say about dependency, however, I am offended by this observation by two researchers, well-known in the field of adult hearing loss:

> Deafness certainly tests a marriage, but the marriage which fails the test may not have been that good anyway. Fortunately, many (so far as we can judge, most) marriages hold firm: the hearing partner helps the deafened one, whose gratefulness binds them closer.[11]

I do not want it to be my gratefulness that binds me closer to Bob. Moreover, I think these researchers underestimate the strains that deafness puts on an otherwise healthy marriage.

> My mother said, "I am helpless." My father said, "Take care of us." I did not ask, "Who will take care of me?" I was alone, walled in their silence and mine.[12]
>
> – *Ruth Sidransky, hearing daughter of (signing) Deaf parents*

Today, people who did not know me before I got my cochlear implant sometimes ask how I managed then. I will start out by insisting that I did hear a bit with my hearing aid. If Bob is present, however, he will invariably interject to say, "She couldn't hear a thing." He will insist (over my objections) that I couldn't hear anything with my hearing aid, and that he could shout my name at me in the same room while my back was turned, yet I would not respond. Bob does not have the same need as I do to believe that I managed fine with my deafness and hearing aid. Maybe his perception is therefore the more objective one. In any case, I'm happy to say, he has a ringside seat to view the slow improvements I have been making in my hearing.

Since I received my implant, my ability to use the telephone and my confidence in understanding what is going on around me have made me feel much less dependent and needy. It's wonderful to be able to call Bob on the telephone and tell him I'll be late for dinner, or to call my friends myself and chat with them. Family conversations are easier for me to follow too, and I feel more a part of things. I have become more able to share Bob's pleasures in folk music and better able to attend and enjoy social gatherings. When I go to folk festivals and concerts with Bob now, he knows that I'm enjoying them too. After I got my implant and learned to hear with it, our socializing increased, and I began to participate more in group conversations. I once asked a friend of Bob's if my speech had improved since I got my implant. She said, "Yes, and there's a lot more of it too!"

I have always, even as a teenager, had a need to squeeze whatever pleasure I could from music, whether it was by listening to a record on the floor with my ears inches from the record player, or by going to small concerts and sitting in the front row with lyric sheets in my hand to try to lipread and follow the printed lyrics. At times I'd eke out some pleasure from these musical events, but often they were just too difficult, and I would be frustrated. Bob's love of music has offered me many opportunities to at least try, and he has been a knowledgeable music mentor. Moreover, we often have music in the house, with friends coming over for a song circle. Since I've received my cochlear implant, we've also started to host house concerts for professional musicians who perform in our living room. I sit in a comfortable chair a few feet away from the performers; for some singers, I request that they bring printed lyric sheets that I can glance at so I can follow the songs more easily. These casual musical events give me an excellent opportunity to enjoy live music.

My parents are no longer alive – they died when Nic was a small child – and I regret that they did not live to see my hearing improve. Leah's pleasure in my newfound ability, however, is gratifying. The first time I called her on the phone, she was thrilled. Unfortunately, I rarely see my brother.

I am, however, still deaf, although usually I function as hard of hearing. Moreover, old habits and personality traits persist, and my deafness can still be a strain on my family. It can still be difficult for me to follow some discussions around the table with Bob and Nic, especially if they are having a quiet or quick conversation, and I have difficulties at social gatherings where people talk all at once.

My deafness is so profound that I expect to miss most of what is being said [in a group conversation]. I let go of the hurt inside, telling myself to relax and watch. I can stay with the conversation in mind and spirit, even if I do not understand most of the words.[13]

– Eve Nickerson, who received a cochlear implant in 1985

Although Bob encouraged me to get an implant and has welcomed my increased independence now that I hear so much more, there has been a subtle shift in the dynamics of our relationship. This change has usually, but not always, been a positive one. Sometimes, in my newfound independence, I can be too quick to shut Bob out. I am still trying to understand how deafness and learning to hear with a cochlear implant have affected my family and my personality, and I don't claim to have fully sorted it out.

Even though he has encouraged me more than anyone to acknowledge and accept my deafness, Bob has been taken aback and often dismayed by the obsessiveness with which I have approached issues relating to deafness and cochlear implants since I first started investigating the devices in 1992. Rather than pushing issues related to deafness to the side in my life, I have now given them a central role. I feel driven to understand deafness better, and to explain it to others. This compulsion has put another strain on our marriage. I have joined the staff of a journal dealing with cochlear implants, I have helped to form a cochlear implant support group in Canada, I have corresponded over the Internet with literally hundreds of people who are deaf, I have attended conferences on deafness, I have spent over a year researching and writing this book. It is as if I am trying to make up for a lifetime of denial.

People who wear cochlear implants need support groups, but so too may their partners. The excitement of getting an implant and the excitement over the changes in the deaf person's life are readily acknowledged. But what of the excitement and changes in the life of the partner? When Bob helped to organize a discussion group for hearing spouses at the 1997 convention of Cochlear Implant Club International in Massachusetts, he found that a recurring complaint of the participants was that they felt isolated from those who were most likely to understand their feelings and needs. They felt lonely. They wanted some acknowledgment of the strains on their own lives and the challenges that both deafness and hearing with an implant presented to them. Many, like Bob, play the role of both coach and cheerleader for their spouses after the surgery, encouraging them in their task of learning to hear, and cheering their successes. But few are able to talk with others in their situation and get the advice or support they may need.[14]

Many of the problems that were voiced at that all-too-short workshop hinted at major problems in the marriages between hearing people and deaf people with cochlear implants. When the hearing spouse says she is having trouble getting her husband to wear his processor all the time, what larger problem is that small one hiding? Is the deafness a problem for her that she is pleading with her husband to do something about? Is the husband stubbornly resisting learning to hear, not wanting to become less dependent on her? Is he struggling with what he is hearing, and unable to ask for help from his audiologist? I can only guess, and hope that they and all the other families in need find support.

Although Bob and Nic and I continue to struggle with the effects of deafness, our love and enjoyment of one another transcends the difficulties, and our sensitivity to what we each are feeling helps us through the rough patches. One of the things that would have helped in this struggle, and that I lacked in the past and am finding only recently, is my own greater acceptance and acknowledgment of my disability. I am still too ready to overcompensate for my deafness, still too quick to become angry at my limitations. I grew up in a small town where there was no support for hearing-impaired children, at a time when deafness was considered shameful. I grew up before the Deaf pride movement, before the Americans with Disabilities Act, before the expression "disabilities activist" was coined. I needed then, and need now too, to acknowledge my deafness and accept it in order to be more comfortable with my limitations, comfortable with asking for help when I need it, and kinder to those in my family who are also coping with my deafness. I'm working on it.

> Learning how to ask for help was difficult for me at first. I did realize, however, that asking for help gives others the opportunity to give help. Through these experiences we learn how to give support to one another. We all need help at one time or another, so I felt that my role in asking for help was a positive one.[15]
>
> – cochlear implant user, Kathy Urschel, who is both deaf and blind, and was the tandem cycling silver medalist in the 1996 Paralympic Games in Atlanta, Georgia

5
BECOMING WIRED
FOR SOUND

It was pleasing to see one of the most desperate of
human calamities [deafness] capable of so much
help: whatever enlarges hope, will exalt courage.[1]
– Samuel Johnson

Whenever I visited my ear, nose, and throat specialist for a checkup, I would ask him, "Is there anything new that can be done for my deafness?" I didn't really expect a positive answer anymore, but in early 1992, he surprised me by saying, "Yes." He suggested that I consult another specialist to determine if I was a candidate for a cochlear implant. I couldn't, however, really allow myself to feel any excitement because over the years I had built up a protective barrier against cures and miraculous remedies. I was even surprised when the receptionist's face lit up with pleasure when the doctor told her to make an appointment for me to obtain a cochlear implant evaluation.

In my younger days, I tried everything from acupuncture and faith healing to hypnotic regression into past lives to "cure" my hearing loss. The implant was certainly a logical move for me.[2]

– cochlear implant user
Paula Bartone-Bonillas

Part of my lukewarm reaction was probably because I had been assessed for a cochlear implant in the past. In the early 1980s I was evaluated for a single-channel implant at the House Ear Clinic in Los Angeles – a leading clinic for the procedure in North America. I had a day filled with several tests and consultations and was hopeful. But at the end of the day, a doctor surveyed the test results and told me that I could do no better with an implant than with my hearing aid. I was terribly crushed. When he said, "The technology will improve, and someday, it may help you," I paid little heed. Now, according to my Toronto doctor, that day had come.

The consultations and tests at the Toronto clinic were spread over several weeks. At a first meeting with the implant surgeon, Dr. Julian Nedzelski, he told me he used a multichannel implant that gave much better results than the single-channel device I had been evaluated for previously. However, he cautioned me that because I had been profoundly deaf for so long, I might obtain nothing more than an improved awareness of environmental sounds and an easier time of lipreading. "If you had been deaf for only a few years," he said, "the situation might be very different." He disappointed me even further by saying the devices weren't meant for music, and most people did not like music they heard with their implants.

> I just love sounds, high sounds, low sounds, staccato sounds, slow sounds. When I sing outside, I feel like my voice is part of Mother Nature.[3]
>
> – Caitlin Parton (at the age of seven), who was deafened at twenty-two months and received an implant at the age of three

Later, after I received my cochlear implant, I listened to Pat Humphries sing "Baptism of Fire." I realized only then that the oboe solo, the sweet thin and high oboe solo within the song, repeated the main melody. How right, how beautiful it sounded, and how obscure it had been in the past. Before I got my implant, I would hear instrumental solos in the middle of a song, and they would just be noise, possibly pleasant noise. I would dutifully clap at the end of an apparently virtuoso solo, without understanding why everyone else was so impressed. I had not realized the solo was singing the melody of the song, sometimes with clever twists and turns. But listening to the oboe solo in "Baptism of Fire," it all fell into place. What a beautiful experience I had missed all those years.

After my meeting with the surgeon, I duly, but with only guarded enthusiasm, proceeded with the tests to determine if I was eligible for an implant. I had a hearing test to determine my thresholds of hearing (they were so high, they were almost impossible to measure), a speech discrimination test to determine how much I could understand with my hearing aid but without lipreading (virtually nothing), and a computer-assisted tomography (CAT) scan to determine if there were any abnormalities in my inner ear (there were none). Then I had a balance test. For that, a technician poured warm and cold water alternately into my ears. She also blindfolded me and spun me around on a chair in a darkened room. (I had no balance problems, but the tests seemed medieval.)

These tests were standard ones to determine if I was a candidate for an implant. Candidates for cochlear implants at that time, in the early 1990s, needed to show on a hearing test that they were profoundly deaf in both ears and obtained little or no benefit from hearing aids. This meant that although they might get some awareness of environmental sounds from them, as I did, they did not achieve significant understanding of speech without lipreading. (By 1998, adults with more hearing were considered as candidates, although children still needed to be profoundly deaf and not benefitting significantly from a hearing aid. Adults who could understand as many as 30% or even 40% of the key words in test sentences without lipreading became eligible at some clinics.) A CAT scan needed to demonstrate that I had a cochlea into which electrodes could be inserted. Some deaf people are born with none or develop bony material within it that might obstruct an implant coil.[4] In the case of adult candidates, normally, they should also have some experience with hearing.

After the tests, I had two interviews with the clinic's audiologist, David Shipp, to discuss what would be involved in the surgery, and what I could expect after my external equipment was turned on. At the first interview, David told me the test results showed that I was indeed a potential candidate for an implant. On my speech dis-crimination tests with my hearing aid and no lipreading, I had scored much lower than the average score of implant users at the clinic who had used their devices for six months. Since my scores were zero or almost zero, I was not difficult to beat. The average score for those implanted at the clinic, six months after their equip-ment was turned on, was 45% of the key words in sentences, with-out lipreading.[5] This score was in line with scores commonly reported at that time.[6] Almost all of the clinic's implant recipients did better than I did with my hearing aid. This was very encourag-ing. I allowed myself to get a little excited.

I wondered how many of the clinic's clients, most of whom had become deaf in adulthood, had acquired my tricks for understanding with very lit-tle actual hearing. I wondered if with all my tricks and strategies and experience with a hearing aid, I might actually be at an advantage over them. I suspected I would, and that these skills might bal-ance the disadvantage I had in being deaf for so long. David was unsure. He could only repeat that my long-term deafness meant I needed to be very modest in my expectations. I could not, for example, be certain that I could ever use the phone in a normal fashion.

A few months after getting my implant, my first telephone conversations were with Bob, over the extension phone. I had to practice with him first, because the embarrassment of using the phone and not understanding at all many years ago had made me apprehensive about the prospect of failing miserably. Initially, I could not understand anything he said. I

Only someone who has been through a lifetime of never being able to use the phone can understand the giddi-ness, the breathtaking sense of triumph I have each time I succeed on the phone. And just today I spent forty-five minutes on the phone chatting with a friend who, like me, has a cochlear implant and had been deaf most of her life.[7]

– Mardie Younglof, who was born profoundly deaf due to maternal rubella, and received a cochlear implant at the age of fifty-three, seven months before sending this excited message out to a dis-cussion group on the Internet

asked him to count from one to ten, and when he got to "six" I had to stop him and say, "Are you sure that was a six?" The *s* and the *x* sibilants sounded so strange over the phone, that his "six" bore no relation to my idea of what six should sound like! But, eventually, I learned not only what "six" sounded like, but also what many other words sounded like over the phone. I made longer more complicated telephone calls (although not always without difficulty) to Bob, then Leah, and then friends, then, finally after about a year, to colleagues at work. When I spoke to Nic on the phone for the first time, he was flabbergasted that I was able to understand what he was saying. It was one of the most liberating experiences I have ever had, to be free to call up anyone in the world and speak to them, just with the press of a few keys.

David brought out an implant system, and showed me the parts of it. It had a gray processor the size of a cigarette pack that I could wear on a belt, or in a pocket, or even in my brassiere. The processor would take a regular or rechargeable battery that would last the day. The microphone was set in a beige earpiece that I would wear over my ear much like a behind-the-ear hearing aid. This microphone would pick up sounds in my environment and send them down to the processor through a thin beige cable I would wear under my clothing.

Inside the processor, the sounds would be quickly converted into electrical codes to indicate which electrodes should be stimulated inside my ear and at what intensity. These coded signals would pass back up the cable to the small wheel-shaped transmitter that would sit behind my ear. This transmitter, which was the size of a quarter, would be held in place by a magnet drawn to the implanted magnet underneath my skin where it was sitting inside the implanted receiver/stimulator case. The signals would cross my skin as radio frequency signals, be decoded by the receiver, and then travel to the electrode array in my inner ear to stimulate the appropriate electrodes. The auditory nerve endings in my inner ear would then sense this stimulation and carry the signals to my brain to be interpreted finally – as sound. This whole cycle was rapid: each cycle took about four milliseconds to complete. Newer, faster systems take even less time. A drawing of my cochlear implant system is at the back of the book on page 232.

David counseled me that the devices did not restore normal hearing and warned that it takes time to achieve good use of an implant. Most clinics are very careful to assess the expectations of the candidate and the family. They may advise against an implant when the candidate (or the family) has unrealistic expectations, or the candidate does not seem personally committed to the procedure. When a well-meaning parent or relative is anxious that the deaf person have the procedure, but the deaf person himself or herself resists or seems not to want the device, alarm signals will likely go off, and the clinic may discourage the deaf person from getting an implant.

In Oliver Sacks's true story, "To See or Not to See,"[8] it was Virgil's fiancée, not Virgil, who wanted the operation to restore his sight. Virgil was happy the way he was. He had organized his life around his blindness, was successful as a massage therapist, and felt no need to have his vision back. He had, after all, been blind for almost all of his life. However, his fiancée was excited about the possibility that he might regain his vision, and he gave in to her wishes. His unfortunate outcome after his operation (he became ill and blind again) is analogous to that of many of the so-called cochlear implant "failures." In many of these cases, the person was a poor candidate to start with. He or she may have been a teenager with poor auditory memory and low motivation to succeed but who had been pressured into getting an implant by parents with unrealistic expectations. Or the deaf person may have expected miraculous performance from the start and given up when that didn't occur.

My surgery, if I decided to go ahead, would be in two stages. At the first surgery, Dr. Nedzelski would insert a "temporary implant" (while I was under a general anesthetic) just outside the round window leading into my inner ear. This single electrode would test the ability of my auditory nerve to deliver electrical impulses to my brain. The Toronto clinic was well known for its studies of the prognostic indicators for successful use of the implant, and the candidacy rules of the clinic dictated that all candidates be tested in this way before a final decision to implant was made. (The clinic has since discontinued this test. Instead, it does a less invasive test under local anesthetic in those cases where the deaf person shows no response on a hearing test.) If the "round window test" went well, David would put me on a list of those to receive a multichannel implant a few months later. There would be no charge to me whatsoever. Everything, right down to the first set of rechargeable batteries, would be covered by Canadian public health insurance. In most countries, government-sponsored or private health insurance pays for cochlear implant procedures and equipment.

The actual surgery for the implant, if my round window test showed I was eligible (and we fully expected that it would), would also be done under general anesthetic. This surgery would last two to four hours. Dr. Nedzelski would make an incision behind my ear and raise a skin flap to expose part of my mastoid bone. He would drill a small depression in the mastoid to hold the receiver (with its magnet) in place and secure it to the bone with sutures. Next, he would carefully slip the electrode array (a slim bundle of electrodes in a single carrier sheath) into the cochlea through a hole drilled just in front of the round window of the inner ear. When he was finished, the doctor would move the skin flap back into place and staple it closed (staples were used in lieu of stitches). I would need to stay in the hospital for two nights to monitor any chance of infection around the incision. The following week, he would remove the staples, and six weeks later, after the incision had healed, David Shipp would fit me with the external equipment and "turn it on." In the meantime, I would be able to wear my hearing aid in the other ear. Some hospitals today do this surgery on an outpatient basis, and the patient goes home the same day. There are even a few surgeons who perform the procedure using a local anesthetic.[9]

Surgeons used the same device as I would receive for children, as well. Although our skulls continue to grow during infancy and childhood, our inner ears are fully grown at birth. Skull growth is accommodated in an implant by slack in the lead from the internal receiver to the electrode array. Therefore, it is not necessary to re-implant children as they grow older.

Dr. Nedzelski had soberly warned me of the risks of surgery (including that of infection, facial paralysis, tinnitus or head noise, and the normal risk of anesthesia). He said the rate for complications was about 10%.[10] I am squeamish about medical procedures and have fainted dead away on more than one occasion from a simple inoculation. I can recall regaining consciousness in various positions, including sprawled on a doctor's couch, sitting upright in a wheelchair, and face down on the floor under a table! However, in this case, I decided not to let the surgery affect my decision. A friend who was a doctor suggested I tell the hospital staff about my squeamishness, since one of her patients had broken her leg after fainting from a needle. My family doctor, who was also a good friend, reassured me that a 10% complication rate for surgery was not high, and that the complications were rarely of a serious nature. The potential to do much better than with my hearing aid was just too attractive to allow my fear of surgery to get in the way. I was starting to get excited. In fact, I was starting to get very excited!

I felt as if I was finally emerging from the basement hearing-aid clinic to which I had been relegated years ago. Then doctors could do nothing for me. Now, I would not only be climbing up from the basement, but I would be speeding up to the highest floors where new science, and new technology, were being dispensed. When I visited the cochlear implant clinic at the Sunnybrook research hospital in Toronto, I soaked up the sharp smells in the hospital's halls. I happily took in all the briskly moving doctors in white coats and delighted in the air of importance, purpose, and excitement that filled the place. It was a heady feeling.

I extracted from David a promise that he would have another person who had received an implant contact me so I could meet someone who wore one. Then I decided to do some research to help me make up my mind. I was still not completely certain I wanted or needed this device. I found it hard to believe that such a seemingly crude electronic device would give me much benefit.

Through the University of Toronto Library, I had access to MED-LINE, a computerized database of medical journal abstracts and citations (see the Resources section at the back of this book). I did a search for articles about cochlear implants and came up with many citations. They showed that virtually all those who received an implant benefitted and could hear better than I could with my hearing aid. Moreover, there were people who had been wearing the implanted devices for more than twenty years with no side effects. In 1992, about 7,000 people around the world had received a cochlear implant. The device that was available to me in Toronto had been approved by the influential U.S. Food and Drug Administration for use in adults in 1985, and in children in 1990. It had become available in Canada at around the same time.

According to my readings, the development of cochlear implants dates back to the late eighteenth century. Alessandro Volta, the Italian physicist whose work on electricity gave his name to a measure of electric current, bravely conducted an experiment on his own ears to see what would happen. He attached two metal rods to active electric circuits and inserted one rod into each ear. Volta reported that he felt something like a blow to his head, followed by the sound of boiling liquid. Apparently, the results were not pleasant, and he didn't repeat his experiment. Although many people who followed him were interested in the use of electrical stimulation as therapy for deafness, many others ridiculed the field and saw it as quackery.[11]

One of the first documented cases of an implant that successfully stimulated the auditory nerve took place in France in 1957. André Djourno, a French electrophysiologist, was looking for a way to stimulate muscles in polio patients. His experiments on animals led him to believe that hearing, too, might be stimulated by a surgically implanted electrode. Djourno teamed up with an otolaryngologist, Dr. Charles Eyries, to implant a deaf man. After they implanted an electrode on his auditory nerve and connected it to a crude signal generator, the deaf man described sounds like crickets or a roulette wheel. He became more aware of environmental sounds and could use his increased awareness of speech rhythm to lipread more easily. In time, he could even distinguish between a few simple words.[12]

In the following years, teams of scientists, engineers and surgeons in France, the United States, Australia, Austria, the United Kingdom, Switzerland, Belgium, West Germany, and other countries worked on developing implant systems. Some scientists, however, were concerned about the safety and efficacy of the procedure and believed that more research on animals was needed before implants were performed in humans. In 1965, Dr. Blair Simmons of California, who in 1964 had implanted the first multichannel implant in a human, submitted a paper on the subject for presentation at a meeting of the American Otological Society. To his dismay, the society rejected his paper as too controversial.[13] (In 1997, papers on cochlear implants made up approximately 10% of the total number of presentations at the 1997 XVI World Congress of Otorhinolaryngology Head and Neck Surgery, in Sydney, Australia.)

Many researchers and surgeons, however, recognized the potential benefit of electrical stimulation and kept implanting deaf people and studying the results, despite the disapproval of some of their peers. Dr. Michael Merzenich, a California neurophysiologist, was skeptical of the devices before he became involved in the field in the 1970s. "What amazed me most," he reflected after he became a convert, "was the absolute love of sound that these patients had. I was surprised by how much useful hearing these early patients gained from use of the [early] primitive cochlear implants."[14]

In succeeding years, surgeons who carried out the procedure demonstrated both its safety and efficacy; neuroscientists experimenting on animals showed that electrical stimulation could actually improve neuronal survival following deafness. However, in 1978, when Professor Graeme Clark performed cochlear implant surgery on his first patient, in Melbourne, Australia, there were still lingering concerns about the safety of the procedure for humans, and the beneficial effects of electrical stimulation were unknown. Jim Patrick, the Australian engineer who helped to develop the device that became the first widely available commercial multi-channel cochlear implant, remembers that Professor Clark's implant team were worried about what would happen when they first turned on their patient's implant.[15] They were apprehensive about the effect electrical stimulation might have on his brain. Professor Clark recalls weeping at the turn on:

> I cried with joy. This was the result of the years of commitment and hope that I had put into leading the project, and also perhaps, some relief that it seemed to be working, when I had been subjected to considerable criticism over the years. It was really a very moving experience for me to know that Rod Saunders was experiencing sound. Particularly when at the first test session he responded to the tune of our national anthem, at the time, "God Save the Queen," by standing up. This pulled out some of the wires and cables. ... I retired to the experimental animal theatre nearby our test room, overcome with emotion. [16]

By 1995, two years after I received my own implant, the U.S. National Institutes of Health Consensus Statement on Cochlear Implants in Adults and Children concluded that "a majority of those [adult] individuals with the latest speech processors for their implants will score above 80 percent correct on high-context sentences, even without visual cues." This conclusion represented an astounding advance over even the 1988 Consensus Statement's weak acknowledgment that "some [users] communicate face-to-face with comparative ease, and even a few (about 5 percent) can carry on normal conversation without lipreading."

Cochlear implants are the first effective artificial sensory organ developed for humans.[17] From Djourno and Eyries's patient in 1957 who perceived sounds in his environment as like crickets to the average implant user today who understands 80% of test sentences without lipreading has been an amazing journey. American audiologist Dorcas Kessler calls it "one of the most rapid advances in medical technology."[18] While early implants may have provided only an awareness of environmental sounds and an improvement in lipreading at best, since the late 1980s, cochlear implants have been providing far more benefit.

The statistics in 1992, when I was doing my initial research, and today still show a wide variation in individual performance. For example, in one study of performance reported in 1997, sixty-one adults were tested on their ability to understand sentences without lipreading six months after their equipment was switched on. Although the average score was 84%, there was a very large range of success. Individuals scored anywhere between 24% and 100%. The range for performance on a more difficult test of monosyllabic words (such as "book" and "ball") without lipreading was even greater. While the average result was an excellent 48%, individual performances ranged between a low of 8% and a high of 90%.[19]

Dr. William House in the United States implanted the first child with an early single-channel device in 1980; Professor Graeme Clark in Australia implanted the first child with a multichannel device in 1985. Long-term speech perception results since then show that a majority of children with multichannel implants develop the ability to understand speech without lipreading. For example, in a set of 100 unselected children and adolescents with multichannel implants in 1995, approximately 60% could understand a significant amount of speech without lipreading.[20] Approximately 30% were able to communicate freely using auditory input alone (with their implant devices). The researchers studying this group, however, were able to account for only 40% of the variance in speech perception scores by connecting individual scores with factors such as age at implantation, duration of profound hearing loss, pre-implant hearing ability, and type of hearing loss. They concluded that "speech perception in children with cochlear implants is inherently unpredictable and/or ... there are factors not included in this analysis that have an important effect." The authors point out that one of these factors may be the home environment.

In another study of a group of thirty-eight children and adolescents, the group was able to understand an average of 32% of the key phrases in sentences presented to them without lipreading, after at least twelve months of experience with their devices.[21] Twenty-one of these children had been born deaf, and fifteen were more than ten years of age when they received their implants. Individual performances ranged between a low of 0% and a high of 94%.

Speech production in children (and adults) can also be positively affected by the use of a cochlear implant. For example, in a detailed study over four years of nine children in Australia implanted at the age of five or younger, all showed a significant improvement in their ability to speak.[22] In the United Kingdom, a study of the first 100 children implanted in the Nottingham program found that five years after receiving their implants, 83% were able to produce speech well enough that they could use it as their primary means of communication.[24]

Today, Dara is seven years old and she attends the same local public school as her brother where she receives excellent itinerant help in her classroom for six hours per week. She is learning French, participates in music, has many friends, and does quite well on the telephone with the help of a speaker phone with volume control. She even had a small speaking role in a made-for-television movie.[23]

– *Shirley and Julian Keller, parents of Dara, whose profound deafness was discovered at the age of eight months, and who received an implant at the age of four*

The same Nottingham study showed that three years after receiving an implant, 85% of the children were able to understand common phrases without lipreading. In the United States, Dr. Mary Joe Osberger reported on the clinical trials as of December 1996 of 181 children implanted with one device.[25] Her report showed that more than half of the younger children were able to understand one or more of ten simple sentences without lipreading six months after receiving their implant. Well over half of the older children were able to understand some of the more difficult monosyllabic words in a test without lipreading.

Although the wide ranges in scores show there are no guarantees for the levels of performance that children (or adults) will achieve, and there are no guarantees of how fast they will achieve these levels, the potential is there for them to achieve modest success and build upon it. Moreover, children who have been deaf from birth or later, but before learning to talk, have shown that they can learn to hear and speak with a cochlear implant. Ninety-eight percent of the children in Dr. Osberger's study were prelingually deaf.

Since the first crude stimulations of the auditory nerve in the 1950s and 1960s, cochlear implants have advanced in at least three major areas: electrode design, signal processing, and miniaturization. I'll describe each of these areas briefly.

Electrodes, the elements that provide direct electrical stimulation inside the cochlea, have developed from single points of crude stimulation to bundled multiple electrodes on an array of wires, the type that I now have. Thanks to the work on biocompatible materials undertaken for cardiac pacemakers and the advances in electronics for the space industry, the implanted electrodes (and implanted receiver/stimulators connected to them) are both safe and highly compact.

Professor Graeme Clark recalls how he mulled over the problem of inserting multiple electrodes into the cochlea. The problem was that the spiral cochlea is not only very small (uncoiled, it is about 32 mm long, and 2 mm in diameter), but it also narrows from its base to its apex. On vacation, Clark found his answer by passing different blades of grass into seashells shaped like the human cochlea. He found that blades of grass graded in stiffness so they were soft and pliable at the tip and stiffer at the other end slipped much more easily into the tightening spirals of the shells.[26] Therein, at the beach, lay the clue to his development of a smooth, tapered sheath for the electrode wires: it would be stiffer at the top and bend easily at the tip, so a surgeon could insert it deeply into the cochlea without breaking it, while inflicting minimal trauma to the delicate inner ear. More recently, electrodes have been developed that are pre-shaped into a spiral. The surgeon inserts these electrodes with a special insertion tool that holds them straight while he is slipping them in, then releases them so they can conform to the shape of the spiral cochlea, to make better contact with surviving neurons in the ear.

The electrode arrays of current cochlear implants[27] bypass the outer ear and middle ear as well as the inner ear's hair cells, to directly stimulate the neurons of the inner ear. The electrodes of auditory brainstem implants (ABIs) go even further: they bypass the entire ear and auditory nerve. For those whose auditory nerves have been severed, for example due to the surgical removal of tumors in neurofibromatosis type 2, cochlear implants will not work. This is because they need an intact auditory nerve to carry signals to the brain from the cochlea, where the surgeon has implanted electrodes. An ABI, however, bypasses the ear and auditory nerve completely; the surgeon places the electrodes directly on the person's auditory brainstem. Aside from the placement of their electrode arrays, the cochlear implant and the ABI are very similar. The ABI electrode array, however, is flat to conform to the brainstem surface, while the electrode array of a cochlear implant is elongated and rounded to fit inside a cochlea.

The ABI is still in an early stage of its development, and only about 150 people had received one by 1997.[28] Generally, success with ABIs is not as good (at least in the short term) as it is with cochlear implants. However, most individuals do benefit, and some achieve pitch discrimination and the ability to understand significant amounts of speech without lipreading – all without the use of the ear or auditory nerve.[30]

The second front on which developers

Doctors and researchers think it quite remarkable ... [that an auditory brainstem implant] can actually produce recognizable sounds. "Recognizable" may not be an accurate term to describe the things I hear ... – often I find it difficult to distinguish a voice from a metal trash can being whacked with a baseball bat! Speaker asks: "How are you today?" I hear: "Whackwack wack wawack?" I answer: "No thank you, I just had one."[29]

– John Petito, an early (1989) single-channel auditory brainstem implant recipient, joking about his hearing ability have made advances in cochlear implant technology is in signal processing. Processing strategies to translate acoustic signals into electrical signals have become progressively more sophisticated, thanks in good part to the studies of human subjects actually using the devices. These people are tested with various strategies and tell researchers what works best, providing information that cannot be obtained from animal studies. One year after I received my own implant, I replaced my processor with an upgraded one in order to run a newer processing strategy. Modern electronics, using advances made in the computer as well as the space industry, has allowed scientists to develop a variety of sophisticated processing schemes to code acoustic signals into useful electrical signals. There have been strategies that extract only specific components of the incoming signal, strategies that stimulate electrodes simultaneously or sequentially, strategies that generate signals in the form of a continuous analogue waveform, or in the form of a series of pulses, strategies that provide different rates at which the electrical signal is refreshed.

Confoundingly, researchers discovered in the 1990s that as a group, individuals with current multichannel processors perform with a similar pattern of results with all these different strategies[31] and their individual performance remains largely unpredictable. There are still very wide variations in results regardless of the device. Variations in individual performance *within* groups of people using the same device are much greater than the overall difference *between* groups that use different current devices.[32]

In recognition of the large differences in people's responses, and the realization that individual differences can be much more important than device differences, the trend in processing strategies has been to give individuals as much flexibility as possible and provide them with a choice of strategy in a single device.

The third major front on which advances have been made is in the size of the external equipment. The early recipients could hear only while they were tethered to the massive computer equipment in the researcher's laboratory. In Australia in 1979, eighteen months after their first fateful cochlear implant surgery, Graeme Clark's team were able to give their first patient a wearable speech processor. It weighed 1.25 kilograms (2.75 pounds) and was the size of a binocular case. The patient, Rod Saunders, wore the processor in a shoulder bag, and its case was improvised from a piece of plastic drainage pipe that had been heated and squashed flat![33] By the 1990s, processors had shrunk to a tenth of the size and weight of that early processor. They became about the size of a cigarette package and weighed around 100 grams (3.5 ounces). Today, most implant manufacturers are at various stages in the development of behind-the-ear processors that can be worn completely at ear level. And at least two device manufacturers are making plans for a totally implantable processor. More and more, implant users are finding it easier to blend in with the crowd.

> *I am at Esalen, a retreat at Big Sur on the coast of California. It is six months after my operation. This is the laid-back home of gestalt therapy and attracts soul-seekers from around the world. As usual at events like this, I am the only deaf person in attendance.*
>
> *It is the final evening of our five-day session and we are all gathered at the simply named "Big House." We are lounging in a circle on the deeply carpeted floor, sitting and leaning on huge velvet cushions. A fire blazes in the fireplace, and I can hear the waves roaring softly in the night just beyond the window. The group has become very close and accepting of one another. I had been assertive during the week and able to frankly discuss my communication needs and limitations as a deaf person. Such an intensive workshop spread out over five days would have been stressful beyond belief in my pre-implant days. But now I am relaxed. I still cannot understand everything, but I do manage to follow enough to stay with the group.*
>
> *A British woman who had been abused as a child and admittedly has trouble with self-acceptance is talking about how having me in the group, with my need to see her face while she was speaking, meant she couldn't hide her face,*

much as she would like to. She covers her mouth with her handkerchief and looks down, to demonstrate how she would like to hide her feelings while she talks. Sensing that I am missing something important as she speaks, I say, "Pardon, I didn't hear that" and the whole room breaks out into laughter. The leader of the group, a psychiatrist, does a backward somersault on the carpet in glee.

Later, another participant, who is visiting from Germany, breaks down and cries. She is so frustrated, she says in slow, heavily accented English, because she cannot understand everything that people are saying. She feels guilty about asking for help, she says. She sobs that it's her fault, not ours, that her English is not good enough, and she cannot follow everything. The group's consciousness level, however, has been raised high. They tell her that the communication problem is not hers alone, but belongs to the whole group. I glow inside.

A few weeks after my meeting with David Shipp to discuss my candidacy, I met, for the first time, someone who wore a cochlear implant. David had asked Lyn Morton to contact me, and we arranged to meet at my house. Lyn came to the house dragging a large shopping bag filled with articles, magazines, and pamphlets. She was a teacher who had suddenly lost her hearing about ten years previously due to meningitis. When I asked her how she liked her implant, she said, "I love it." It was clear that the device was a huge help for her; her sudden deafness in adulthood had allowed her to develop very few of my lipreading and coping skills. She showed me how she wore her processor (in a black nylon pouch on her skirt belt) and showed me the brown coiled transmitter hidden by her hair behind her ear. There was a beige cord snaking down from it inside her clothing to the processor. Frankly, it looked awkward and uncomfortable.

After Lyn left, I went through her shopping bag and devoured the printed materials inside. One magazine that was especially interesting was *CONTACT*, which I learned was the quarterly journal of a support organization called Cochlear Implant Club International. It had articles about current research and personal experience stories of people with implants. (Many of the quotations throughout this book are ones I have taken from CONTACT articles.) One article listed electronic mail addresses for people who were prepared to exchange e-mail with others. I sent a message to Larry Orloff in Massachusetts, the editor of the magazine, and we struck a common chord immediately. Late one night, when I could not sleep because of all the thoughts about deafness and cochlear implants running through my head, I sent an e-mail message to Joanne Syrja in California. I had taken her e-mail address from an article she published in CONTACT about her experiences leading up to her cochlear implant surgery. She too had grown up with a hearing impairment, and it seemed from the article that we had a lot in common. There was an e-mail response waiting for me the next morning, and after we found we indeed had a great deal in common, we became close friends.

These e-mail friendships were important, because I desperately needed to talk to others in a similar position. The information my surgeon and audiologist gave me could answer only a few of the many questions I had. Would the surgery be painful? How visible would the shaved patch of my scalp be before my hair grew back? What would it be like to get turned on? How would it sound? Would it be too loud? Would the sounds hurt my head? Would it all be stressful? What could I do to learn to use the new sounds? Would I be able to go into work immediately after getting turned on? I had hundreds of questions! The Internet proved to be a tremendous help in expanding my network of connections to include implant users around the world who could answer those questions. Larry and Joanne and the many other people I met online were to give me warm support and mentoring throughout my voyage, and remain good friends today. Larry and Joanne were also the first close friends that I made who were deaf. In 1993, shortly after I received my implant, I joined them on the editorial staff of CONTACT.

There is a wonderful bonding that often takes place between deaf people with cochlear implants or those who are candidates for the procedure. We click. We understand as those who are hearing cannot, the thousands of barriers that deafness throws at us within a hearing milieu. And we have in common a desire to overcome those difficulties as best we can in order to live our lives within a hearing environment. In many cases, we have been traveling through deafness seemingly alone, sometimes passing as hearing. Now thanks to our shared excitement about this small device, we have finally come together and realized we were not traveling alone.

While I was still trying to decide if I wanted to proceed, I took Nic, who was then seventeen years old, and Bob with me to a local meeting of a cochlear implant users' group. I knew I would be leaning heavily on them for support after I got my cochlear implant, so I wanted to involve them early. Nic and Bob were starting to share my excitement and were quite willing to come along. But after listening to one woman talk about how she could not hear as well after she bumped her head on a kitchen cabinet door, and others complain about crackling cords and broken parts, and seeing the way in which many cochlear implant users still struggled to follow what was being said, Nic's enthusiasm waned. "It's up to you, Mom," he said, "but I think you're doing okay without the implant. You're doing better than most of the people who have it. Why take a chance on this?" I could see his point: most of the adults were late-deafened and had poor lipreading skills. Many seemed to have trouble conversing in the noisy room before and after the meeting. But, as I told him, I sometimes only appeared to be managing well. I reminded him of his and his father's chagrin (as they told me later) at my confidently answering queries put by someone in the audience at the meeting. Only both times, my answers were to the wrong questions. I hadn't heard the questions properly, even though I thought I had. He said, "Oh, you're always doing that."

I understood Nic's surprise at my desire to do something about my deafness, and his feeling that I was managing just fine the way I was. A part of me also resisted the idea of an implant, resisted the suggestion that I was not coping well enough with deafness. I need-ed to feel I was managing just fine with my hearing aid and my tricks and strategies. I even felt a flicker of annoyance when people told me I would "hear again" after I received an implant. I thought I heard then. I was like a blind person who insists that she's fine and can manage quite well, thank you. But when you look closer you realize she is covered with bruises and welts from bumping into things and doesn't even know she is hurt, so determined is she to keep moving.

At a second meeting with David, I brought Bob so that he could ask any questions he had. David patiently explained to Bob the nature of the surgery, and the equipment I would be wearing, and how most implant users do much better with a cochlear implant than I did with a hearing aid. He said it would take time for me to get adjusted to the new sounds, and I would need Bob's help. Bob listened carefully, and when David asked if he had any questions, there was a long pause. Then Bob said, "What would happen if two people each got a cochlear implant, and they went to bed together? Would their implanted magnets make them repel each other?"

When I visited the surgeon for a second meeting, I told him I had decided to go ahead. I felt I had nothing to lose (especially if we implanted the ear that wore no hearing aid), and possibly much to gain. It was exhilarating to think I might actually become less deaf. It meant a possibility of rebirth and transformation, and how could I not be excited (and scared) by such a possibility?

Dr. Nedzelski asked me which ear I wanted implanted. Only one ear is normally given an implant, with the other ear left available for future, more advanced interventions. Because inserting the implant in the inner ear can destroy the remaining hearing in that ear,[34] and because I did not want to give up my hearing aid and all the com-plex adaptations I had made over the years to hearing with it, I asked that we implant the other ear. It had worn a hearing aid for a few years when I was a teenager, but since then, had been unable to wear one. When I put a hearing aid in that ear, I could make no sense of the sounds I received. Moreover, I could not tolerate amplification in it, and developed tinnitus if I wore the volume control turned up to anything past a uselessly low level. Because I had no guarantees that I would hear much better with an implant, and because of my fear of losing what little hearing ability I had developed, I chose the otherwise useless right ear to receive an implant. In retrospect, I might have done better to have chosen the ear that had more experience with sound and better discrimination. Moreover, the surgery seems not to have destroyed my residual hearing. When I slip a hearing aid into my implanted ear now, there seems to be no change – I can hear as well (or rather as poorly) with it now as I could before my surgery.

Before I left the clinic, I signed a form saying I wanted to proceed even though I understood that there were no guarantees as to my performance after surgery and that the range of benefit for individuals was very great. The form described average performance and said in bold letters, "Regardless of how well cochlear implant users do with their devices, implants do not restore normal hearing." I was prepared to do whatever I could to give myself a break, and cut myself some slack, however little it might be.

It is a year after I received my implant, and I am driving home from the hospital after visiting a woman who has just received her own cochlear implant. She had only been deafened for a short time in adulthood before her surgery. I think about how she had been so outraged that the hospital had not known how to deal with a deaf person. She had been indignant that the nurses had not supplied her with a special phone for the deaf (a TTY), that they had not understood without being told that she needed to lipread. When she told me about these things, I had been sympathetic, but I had not shared her indignation. I had held back. In the car, thinking back to her litany of how unfair things had been, I find myself crying uncontrollably. Yes, deafness is unfair. But there was such a huge difference between this woman's righteous anger and expectations, and my years of suppressing my anger, of taking the onus on myself to change my environment so my deafness could be accommodated. I felt torn between the right-ness of her indignation and expectations, and my own habitual approach that said I could expect nothing unless I asked for it, and that I should ask for help only if I couldn't manage by myself. The gap in expectations between this woman, deafened in adulthood, and myself, growing up deaf and powerless, is huge. And now, I find myself crying for all the times when I felt powerless, when my needs were unrecognized, and when I couldn't ask for what I needed.

I had my round window stimulation test in September of 1992. The time for the surgery kept getting pushed back because of more urgent surgeries that day. I developed a tremendous headache, probably because I went for about eighteen hours without food or drink. In fact, the headache is the main thing I remember. While I was under a general anesthetic, the surgeon made an incision in my eardrum and slipped a single electrode through it to sit at the round window to my inner ear.

The morning after the surgery, I dressed and walked down to the lab to have David test the electrode. The test took about five minutes and simply determined my thresholds for electrical stimulation and my ability to distinguish between a few different frequencies. For some frequencies, I could actually feel the electrode vibrating. For some, I could feel a quivering sensation in my tongue. (Neither of these things later happened with my cochlear implant.) The sounds were strange beeps and buzzes, and nothing to be thrilled about. David pronounced himself satisfied

When I had my promontory stimulation test [similar to the author's round window stimulation, to determine the viability of the auditory nerve], after having heard nothing at all for forty-one years, I couldn't be sure at first if I was feeling or hearing something. When the doctor turned the sound up too loud, it went right through my body and felt like an orgasm.[35]

– *Nancy Hoffmann, who became totally deaf from meningitis at the age of six* with my thresholds and sent me to Dr. Nedzelski to have the electrode removed from my ear. I went home that day, feeling far better than I did when I went into the hospital with my terrible headache.

I had now satisfied the final criterion for candidacy and was put on the list for implant surgery. This was to be several months away. I continued to talk to people with implants and to do research. I was even on the point of writing the very next day to an audiologist in California to discuss whether I should wait for an alternative implant device to become available in Toronto, when I got word that my surgery had been moved forward and would take place in a few weeks, on May 18.

When there is a choice, choosing between implant device brands can be difficult. Moreover, my implant surgeon made it clear at my first visit that the device he surgically implanted would stay in my head until I died, and that he would not remove it to replace it with another device if a superior one came along. So, my decision would need to be a very careful one. In 1993, there was only one brand of device available to me in Toronto. Today, there are two or three. But even in 1993, there were reports of great success with a seemingly more advanced device that was then undergoing clinical trials in the United States. Should I have waited for that device to become available? I don't know. At the time, it seemed there was no conclusive proof of superiority. The range in performance continued to be wide, regardless of the device. I was like a potential computer buyer trying to decide whether to get a computer now or wait for the new more advanced version just around the corner. I decided not to wait, but to jump in and take advantage of the technology available to me at that time, and hope that all or most of the updates would be to parts outside my head.

I realized very shortly after my surgery, however, that this would not be my last implant operation. I remember sitting at my desk, with the staples from my recent surgery still in place, reading a transcript of a talk given the previous week by the California audiologist to whom I had been about to write. She was talking about device differences and the need for a very fast refresh rate for some of the newer processing strategies. When I finally understood that my implanted stimulator and electrode array would be too slow to run these strategies, I had a good cry. Then I decided to do the very best I could with what I had. I also resolved to keep my eye on new developments and jump in yet again when it was time to get a second implant in my other ear.

Once the date for the actual surgery was set, I was less apprehensive about it than I had been for the round window test. I more or less knew what to expect, and much of my fear of the surgery was now gone. I also knew that when I regained consciousness, I would be lying in a bed, not under a table! On the day of my surgery, I wore my glasses into the operating room, so I could lipread, and kept my hearing aid on in the ear that was not to be implanted. I wore the hearing aid as much to avoid any possibility that the surgeon might accidentally implant my "good" ear as to help me hear.

Dr. Nedzelski came out of the operating room twice to the hallway where I was lying to speak to me briefly and squeeze my hand before I was wheeled in for the operation. Each time, he asked, "Which ear?" and I would say, "The right ear, the one that is not wearing the hearing aid." The surgery lasted about three hours and was uneventful. The resident surgeon who spoke to me later said it was one of the smoothest insertions he had ever seen, and the full length of the electrode array had gone in with no problem.

I felt quite well after I was wheeled down from the recovery room and felt very little pain. I had a huge bandage wrapped over my ear and around my head. It made me look like pictures I had seen of Vincent van Gogh after he cut off his ear, although I hoped that mine was still under the bandage. After reassuring Bob and Nic and my sister and brother-in-law, who were waiting for me in my

Being in the hospital was a real drag. A lot of the nurses don't know you're deaf and they try to talk to you, or worse yet, come running in telling you the phone is ringing and to pick it up![36]

– *Chris Arcia, who received a multichannel auditory brainstem implant in 1993* hospital room, that I was fine, I threw up. I slept fitfully that night because my ear was uncomfortable to sleep on. The next morning, I felt woozy and threw up once more when I tried to walk to the washroom. But then I felt better, and even hungry. After a second night in the hospital, I went home to finish reading the pile of books I had brought with me. I felt amazingly well, with just some numbness in my skull, and a little weakness from the general anesthetic.

The next week I had my staples removed, and the following week, I was back at work after a two-week absence. I could even comb my longish hair over the small shaved patch of my scalp behind my ear, so there was no outward sign at all of my surgery. I felt just fine.

Now began the wait for the turn on. This was to be the most difficult part of the whole procedure. I waited for that day with huge excitement. I thought of very little else in the six weeks between the surgery and the day my equipment would be switched on. I was turned inside out emotionally. I kept telling myself and everyone else that my expectations were very low. But if that was the case, why was I so feverishly excited? I spoke of little else, boring everyone with whom I came into contact. The possibility of a change in my life was just so overwhelmingly exciting that I could think of nothing else. There existed the possibility not only of a transformation, but also, although I did not realize it then, the possibility of coming through the experience to a deeper understanding of my deafness and its role in my life.

Baptism of fire, all happening within
Illusions burn like tall grass
In the wild and reckless wind
And now they're coming down around me
And I am rising up
Like a great bell resurrected
Ringing loud and true
The only way out is through[37]

A LIGHTNING ROD
FOR THE DEAF
CULTURE

*Disabled is a label that historically has not belonged
to Deaf people. ... When Deaf people discuss their
deafness they use terms deeply related to their language, their past, and their community.*[1]
– Carol Padden and Tom Humphries

There are those who see deafness not as a disability, the way I see
it, not as something to be avoided or "worked on" with therapy, but rather as something for them to welcome and relish.
Although deafness, often from birth, has not been a choice for
them, if given the hypothetical choice of being deaf or being hearing, some of them say they would choose to be deaf. Instead of rail-
ing at the isolation that deafness engenders in a hearing milieu,
deaf people who sign have joined together into a close-knit cultural community of the Deaf.

Deaf culture and capital-*d Deaf* are the terms used to describe the
community of signing deaf people, as opposed to those who are only
audiologically (lower-case-*d*) deaf like me. Although I am deaf, and
have some things in common with all other deaf people, because I
do not use sign language, I am not a member of the Deaf culture.

Many members of this culture share the view that deafness is not a disability, but a cultural affiliation and an accentuation of the sense of vision. Some Deaf people, although they identify with the signing Deaf culture, are in fact only hard of hearing (rather than profoundly deaf). What brings the Deaf together into a "culture" is not their degree of deafness, but their common use of sign language, and their shared values and norms developed and fostered at residential schools for the deaf, and Deaf clubs and associations.

American Sign Language, or ASL as it is called, is a language with its own lexicon and grammar. Used throughout North America, it developed almost 200 years ago from a combination of French Sign Language and indigenous American signs. It is not a gestural form of American English, or a pidgin version of English; nor are Danish, Russian, Israeli, or Chinese Sign gestural or pidgin forms of their corresponding languages.[2] William Stokoe's paper, "Sign Language Structure,"[3] described ASL systematically for the first time in 1960, but without naming it. In 1965, *A Dictionary of American Sign Language*, which Stokoe edited with his colleagues Carl Croneberg and Dorothy Casterline, further codified the language and was notable for including a description of the social and cultural characteristics of the signing deaf. This marked the first time that Deaf culture was formally described as such. The term is now used to describe not only those who use ASL, but signing Deaf in countries around the world.

In many countries in the past (and even some today too[4]), the deaf have been considered ineducable. For example, in England although education for children was made compulsory in 1876, it was not until 1893 that deaf children were required to attend school. In Europe, up until the middle of the eighteenth century, deaf mutes were not even recognized as persons by the law. They were unable to marry or inherit property or receive an education (unless they managed somehow to be trained to speak). Because they were unable to speak, they were considered less than human. The word "dumb" carries the meaning of being unable to speak, but also of being stupid. The legacy of the term "deaf and dumb" is still with us.

When we moved to Toronto I saw signing deaf people for the first time. They were standing in a group on a subway platform waiting for a train. Around them, people were staring passively into space. The Deaf people, on the other hand, were gesturing animatedly with their hands, and wrinkling their noses and twisting their faces. I was fascinated and could not tear my eyes away. My eleven-year-old self was embarrassed on their behalf for this public show of emotion and gesticulating. I had, after all, been taught not to use my hands even to point in public. I remember feeling embarrassed for them, and embarrassed for me too, because I knew that I was like them in my deafness.

Hearing people, even today, may misunderstand and even misdiagnose deaf people and place them in institutions for the mentally retarded.[5] In the larger society, the inability of the Deaf (and deaf) to communicate in the same terms as the rest of the community is often interpreted as a sign of low intelligence. Even though I speak, and do not use sign language, all my life I have experienced times when I have been treated as if I were not too bright because I did not understand what was said. "Sign here. You write your name here. With your pen. On this line," the bank teller tells me in baby-talk, pointing at a deposit slip where I am to sign. As soon as she learned I was deaf, my perceived intelligence plummeted.

It doesn't help that a 1993 U.S. study of the reading comprehension of seventeen-year-old deaf and hard-of-hearing adolescents showed a median score corresponding to Grade 4.5. These were youths in programs that received special education services of some sort. The median score for those who were in residential and day schools for the deaf was even lower. It was at the level of Grade 3.8.[6] Some critics blame the low achievement levels of the deaf on the large chunks of school time many of them may spend learning to speak when, the critics say, they do not need to if they have sign language.

Whenever people exclaim over my good speech (for someone so deaf), and my achievements (again, for someone so deaf), I squirm.

I don't need sound for communication now. I have a collection of skills and options, including professional sign language interpreters and real-time captioning. I have a social circle that accepts deafness and can communicate with me. I have to think that I became deaf as part of a Grand Plan, and that is what I am meant to be. It has had its difficulties, but it has also brought my life some of its greatest joys and successes.[7]

– Kathryn Woodcock, in 1993 explaining why she did not want a cochlear implant

It sometimes seems to me they are saying that the norm for someone as deaf as I am is very low, and that it is surprising I have achieved so much. I feel like a fraud when I am praised for not being like the stereotype of a deaf person. I know that there are a huge number of factors that determine how we, the deaf, make our way through life. How deaf we are, when we became deaf, the cause and progress of our deafness, our family and larger social milieu, our teachers, the expectations of those around us, our personalities – all these and many more factors determine how "well" we do (or how hearing-like we are). Moreover, there are high-achieving Deaf artists and authors and scholars, about whom most hearing people, safe in their stereotypical thinking about the deaf, know nothing. And even those who are not ostensibly achieving great things may still be living satisfying and full lives no less than those of the hearing.

The Deaf have built up around their different way of communicating, a formalized, rich language of signs, different schools (often residential), a different attitude toward personal contact (hugs are commonplace greetings), and a directness that polite hearing company may find uncomfortable. (A friend of mine was told bluntly by a Deaf woman that she was fat. Period.) The Deaf have turned their adaptation to something otherwise negative, deafness, into a way of life within which they can function comfortably. They have turned what others may regard as a physical deficit into something even desirable to have, in the midst of a hearing society that often does not understand them.

In the early 1990s, in Toronto, members of the signing Deaf culture, cochlear implant users, and professionals met to discuss cochlear implant programs and present their views on implanting children. A Deaf woman stood up to express her opposition to cochlear implants in children. She was using sign language, and an interpreter voiced what she was saying. She did not have a child, she signed, but if she had one and it was born hearing, she would find some way to make the child deaf. The audience gasped. This was my own first inkling of a new way of looking at deafness.

In some Deaf families, the birth of a deaf child is cause for a special party, just because the child is deaf. In the wonderfully bittersweet French documentary, *Le Pays des Sourds (In the Land of the Deaf),*[8] one of the characters says ruefully that when his daughter was born, he was hoping for a deaf child and was disappointed when she was born hearing. After a pause, he gives a Gallic shrug and says that he still loves her.[9]

Many of us who get cochlear implants hate deafness with a passion and want more than anything else to be hearing. Those in the signing Deaf culture, on the other hand, have learned what we have been unable to learn: how to love their deafness, embrace it, and yes – accept it fully.

> I lived in the totally deaf world for eight years and have no desire to return. They were eight miserable years. It is so difficult for me to understand how anyone who has tasted the hearing world could ever be happy without sound or could deprive a child the right to grow up experiencing what sound is like. I identify sound with "living." If they had told me they would have had to destroy my implant to keep me alive [when I had my heart attack], I am not sure I would have allowed it.[10]
>
> – *cochlear implant user Gordon L. Nystedt*

Two major milestones in the history of Deaf culture were the International Conference of Teachers of the Deaf held in Milan in 1880, and in 1988, the Deaf President Now movement at Gallaudet College, at that time the only university in the world exclusively for deaf people. The first event marked a low point in the history of the culture, the second a high point. At the international conference in

Milan, educators from around the world resolved that speech was superior to signing in the education of deaf children. Sign language, which was until then commonly used in teaching the deaf, was to be discouraged or forbidden in schools for the deaf. Instead, oralism became the approved method of instruction. Moreover, the educators further polarized the emotional oral/sign debate by resolving that "pure oralism" was preferred over any combination of spoken language with signs. As a result of the resolutions at Milan, oralism was promoted, and deaf teachers became effectively excluded from teaching deaf children in schools for the deaf in many countries around the world.

The second milestone, the American Deaf President Now movement, happening 108 years later, was indirectly an attempt to reverse some of the effects of the conference in Milan. The movement sought to install a deaf president at Gallaudet in place of the hearing president the college's board of trustees had selected. The chair of the board, defending the board's choice, had declared that "deaf people are not ready to function in a hearing world." The students and many others, incensed by the choice and by the insensitive remark, organized demonstrations and a strike at the college. Widespread media coverage elevated Deaf pride and brought an awareness of Deaf culture into mainstream hearing society. The campaign was successful (but only to some extent, as the Deaf candidate lost to the deaf one), and I. King Jordan, who had been deafened as a young adult, was appointed the first deaf president of Gallaudet.

In another manifestation of Deaf pride, the Deaf have united around opposition to a procedure that gives hearing to carefully selected deaf individuals. Opposition to cochlear implants, especially in children, has become a rallying point for Deaf culture and a lightning rod for their dissatisfaction over the way hearing society views the Deaf. Most members of the Deaf culture would not be considered candidates for

> When I first heard about the cochlear implant, I felt hurt inside. Did that mean people didn't like deaf people?[11]
>
> – Charlene LeBlanc,
> then vice president of the
> Ontario Association for the
> Deaf, 1994

the procedure because immersion in the hearing world is generally an important prerequisite of success with a cochlear implant. Nonetheless, many Deaf people view the procedure as an insult and a threat.

I understand this opposition with regard to the Deaf asserting that their lives are not so terrible as hearing people looking at their world from the outside may think. Strangely, I even find myself, almost against my will, extending my empathy and understanding to their opposition to cochlear implants. I find myself comprehending it on a level where my own pain about deafness resides. So I understand the feeling behind even this statement opposing implants, which was issued by a Canadian Deaf association:

> The Deaf community views the use of surgery which pre-vents a child from developing within the [Deaf] cultural minority to be a form of genocide prohibited by the United Nations Treaty on Genocide. Cochlear implants on young healthy deaf children is a form of communi-cation, emotional and mental abuse.[12]

The press release, which went on to suggest that cochlear implan-tation may also constitute "ethnic purification," was written during a period when the civil war in the former Yugoslavia was raging, and each night my television screen showed the grisly and graphic reports about the war's so-called "ethnic cleansing," in which one group tried to eradicate another so as to make the whole "pure." The reverberation of the phrase "ethnic purification" was terrible. In spite of the pleasure I share in Deaf pride after growing up ashamed of my deafness, in spite of how I ache to see all deaf people better understood and accepted in mainstream society, I find myself sad-dened and even embarrassed by the arguments some Deaf advocates use to defend their opposition to implants.

While not all those signing deaf people who are members of the Deaf culture are opposed to cochlear implants in children, many of the organizations that represent them are. The National Association of the Deaf in the United States, *Sourds en Colère* (Angry Deaf) in France, the Canadian Association of the Deaf, the Swedish Deaf Association, the German Deaf Association, the Australian Association of the Deaf, and other Deaf associations have all opposed cochlear implants for children.

Deaf organizations may state that adults who choose to have this procedure have the right to do so, and target their opposition primarily at implants in children. There is often, however, an indirect condemnation of adult implant users. The Canadian Cultural Society of the Deaf, for example, in its position paper on the use of cochlear implants[13] says, "Although cochlear implantation may have some value as a biotechnical assistive hearing device for postlingually deafened adults, its effectiveness is altogether too limited to justify its exorbitant cost." It goes on to chide hearing society that "deafness requires acceptance by the society's mainstream, rather than a ceaseless quest for medical and technological solutions."

> When the Chinese revolution came, the cadres unbound the feet of the women and forced them to run through the streets on their putrid stubs. Is that the future that awaits implanted children? For a revolution of consciousness and pride is surely taking place in the Deaf community.[14]
>
> – *Judith Treesberg, writing in a publication of the National Association of the Deaf*

The cost of the implant procedure (about $40,000 U.S. including surgery, the device, and follow-up care) is no higher, in fact, than it is for many other surgical procedures that can enhance the quality of life for the recipient. Reporting in the *American Journal of Otolaryngology*,[15] Robert Wyatt and his colleagues pointed out that the cost-effectiveness rating of the cochlear implant is above that of many other common procedures such as defibrillator implants to regulate the heart's rhythm and knee replacement surgery.

Moreover, in those cases where it could be helpful, there is a cost associated with not getting a cochlear implant. It is far more costly to educate a child in a residential school for the deaf than in a regular class or in a self-contained class for deaf children in a regular school.[16] Moreover, a lifetime dependence on sign language inter-preters to interpret at meetings with hearing doctors, lawyers, teach-ers, and others is expensive, whereas adults with cochlear implants are likely to manage independently in these situations. This is not to say that those who need these schools and services should not get them because of their expense. I mention the costs here only to point out the weakness of any arguments against cochlear implants based on financial considerations.

In Canada, where the public health-care system completely cov-ers the cost of the cochlear implant procedure, the Canadian Association for the Deaf in 1994 urged the Canadian government to halt government funding for all implants for a two-year period while a study of the safety and efficacy of the procedure was carried out. After undertaking a brief investigation of the matter, the Canadian government was unconvinced of the need for a moratori-um. The minister of National Health and Welfare, in her decision not to accede to the request for a moratorium, said, "The peer reviewed literature overwhelmingly supports the safety and efficacy of these medical devices as a rehabilitative solution for the pro-foundly deaf. A full range of results has been observed, from mod-erate to excellent. However even with moderate results patients greatly benefit from the implants."[17]

In the United States, the National Association of the Deaf (NAD) has complained[18] that they should have been consulted by the Food and Drug Administration (FDA) when the regulatory agency first investigated the efficacy and safety of cochlear implants. If given the opportunity, the NAD said, it would have described the cultural advantages of just staying deaf. At its 1996 convention in Portland, Oregon, the NAD passed a mandate to renew efforts to repeal the FDA ruling that approved implants for children in 1990. In 1997, however, when the FDA reviewed clinical results in chil-dren using a new cochlear implant system, they did hear the NAD arguments, yet unanimously approved the new device.

In frustration, some American Deaf culture advocates have called for legislation that would eliminate the right of parents to implant

> As beneficiaries of the cochlear implant and as victims of prejudice and misunderstanding, we have been given an opportunity for a hearing ear and understanding heart.[19]
>
> – *Larry Orloff*

a deaf child under the age of eighteen. The cultural gap between hearing and deaf on one side, and the Deaf on the other, sometimes appears unbridgeable.

For a long time, I had looked with envy on the apparent easefulness of life in a completely signing world, in a Deaf community. When the strain of lipreading and passing as hearing got to be too much for me, I would cast fond glances at those who seemed to have found a less complicated, easier life in the Deaf culture. Their acceptance of deafness, their surrender to it, were seductive. But I knew that I could not break into the Deaf culture even if I wanted to. I was not a fluent signer – the signs I had learned as an adult at night school were primitive. I had not grown up signing, not gone to Deaf schools, and so would always be suspect in any Deaf group. There was little acceptance within the Deaf culture for a deaf adult who came to signing late in life. Using hearing aids was frowned on. Using one's voice was discouraged. "Thinking-hearing" was a pejorative term. I was stuck: I was not hearing, but I could not be part of the Deaf world either.

An argument used frequently against the implant is that it precludes taking advantage of future developments that might give a child even better hearing. Several Deaf culture organizations have noted the possibility of damage being done to the cochlea as a result of inserting an electrode array. The surgery, they say, is therefore wrong because it prevents children from benefitting from interventions in the future that could, for example, regenerate inner ear hair cells.[20] It is true that implantation may cause physical trauma to the cochlea that can destroy some or all residual hearing. Implant teams routinely warn candidates and their families of this possibility. The residual hearing is typically so poor and provides so little functionality in *bona fide* candidates, however, that this possible destruction is not generally a serious consideration. Moreover, surgeons implant only one ear at a time, generally leaving the second ear available for future developments such as ear hair cell regeneration.

Deaf culture opponents of cochlear implants also say that parents should let the child grow up to make the decision to get an implant himself or herself later as an adult. However, waiting for the child to be old enough to make an implant decision on his or her own is self-defeating – many studies have found that the earlier the operation takes place following the diagnosis of deafness, the greater the likelihood of success. There is, for example, a crucial early period for the development of language – any language, signing or oral. Once this period has passed, it is very difficult or even impossible for a child to catch up.

Speaking about the ethical considerations surrounding the decision by parents to implant or not implant their child, or to delay a decision, J. D. McCaughey, a former member of the Medical Research Ethics Committee, National Health and Medical Research Council in Australia, says, "In this case postponement could be a dereliction of duty on the part of the parent. ... It is the clear duty of parents, if offered the opportunity, to make a firm decision one way or another, and live with the consequences, which are considerable either way."[22]

> If my child steers towards oralism and she wants the implant, then so be it. I just feel it should be the individual's choice. If my child had the implant, and it wasn't successful, would she resent me for trying to change her? I guess that is my real worry.[21]
>
> – *Sarah Butler, mother of a deaf child*

I am flying home from a conference in California. I have told the stewardess that I would not be able to understand the flight announcements and asked her to come to my seat to repeat anything important for me. To my surprise, she comes down the aisle to tell not just me, but also the woman sitting beside me what the announcements were. Moreover, the woman beside me is communicating with the stewardess by writing

notes. I realize that she too is deaf and strike up a written con-
versation with her. She writes back to me that she is an English
professor at Gallaudet University. She tells me she is not wear-
ing her hearing aid because of the loud noise of the airplane,
and when she is without her hearing aid, she cannot use her
voice very well. (Neither can I without my implant turned on.
I screech.) So she writes notes instead. She tells me happily
that she is engaged to be married and that her fiancé is also
deaf. I ask if there is a chance their children will be deaf. She
says yes, they might, because her fiancé's deafness is heredi-
tary. "It's not so bad to be deaf today, though," she writes.
"There are all kinds of things like TTYs and captioning for deaf
people."

I write, "What about cochlear implants? Would you get a
cochlear implant for your child?"

"No, I would wait and let the child decide when he was
about eighteen years old."

"But, by then, wouldn't it be too late for a deaf person to
learn good speech?" I ask. She thinks for a moment.

"I'd never thought of that," she writes.

To get a better understanding of the arguments against cochlear
implants, I conducted a magazine interview in 1994 with a Deaf
culture spokesperson.[23] Gary Malkowski was an elected member of
the provincial parliament in Ontario, Canada, and a prominent
advocate in the North American Deaf culture. He was adamantly
opposed to cochlear implants in children.

I sent Gary several interview questions, asking him about himself
and his views on cochlear implants. A long typed reply came back,
outlining Gary's painful experiences in schools, even in a residential
school for the deaf, where he could not use signs. He remembered
being strapped on his hands whenever he tried to sign. He talked
about the liberation he felt when he first was exposed to an almost
completely signing environment at Gallaudet College in
Washington. "I began to discover who I really was, and to identify

my peer group. I had a right to be Deaf, and therefore to the language of my Deaf culture and its accompanying history. In short, I gained back my self-respect."

Gary said he was in favor of parents making a choice about an implant on behalf of their child. "But I must be honest," he said. "It touches me in a personal way since it brings up memories of my own childhood experiences with oral/aural training. ... This training did not foster self-esteem, but destroyed it. This has permanently left me with negative feelings about my speech and hearing. I have no desire to see other deaf children experience what I did."

This, I realized, was the key to understanding his opposition. Gary was, with all the best intentions in the world, projecting his own old childhood hurt onto the children who get cochlear implants. I recognized in Gary's empathy for deaf children the source of my own empathy for the Deaf culture, and my tolerance for their sometimes outrageous opposition to cochlear implants. We both know that it is painfully hard to grow up deaf in a hearing milieu.

But I didn't think Gary realized how much easier it is now for children who have far more help from cochlear implants than hearing aids were ever able to deliver. I called him to discuss his response, and we talked on the TTY. I tried to explain to him that the quantity and range of sounds that I, a profoundly deaf adult, received with my cochlear implant were enormously greater than what I had been accustomed to with a

> There is a misconception about the "extensive rehabilitation" that CI children receive. [My daughter] was not involved in "formal and structured drills and lessons" at all times. ... Rather, the goal of everything during the course of her day was to teach her language. Thus a trip to the beach would mean that her mother would talk to her about the sand, the sun, the water, etc. ... They would talk for hours about everything. ... As a result of the time they spent together talking to each other, they now have an extremely close relationship.[24]
>
> – Rick Apicella, whose daughter was diagnosed as profoundly deaf at the age of thirteen months and received an implant at two and a half

hearing aid. I felt certain that if I had been given a cochlear implant when my hearing loss became profound in my early teens, I would have coped more easily with deafness than I did using my hearing aids. Moreover, modern-day auditory-verbal therapy that encourages the deaf child's self-esteem has little in common with the drill-type auditory training Gary underwent as a child. I was unable to convince him.

Gary talked about "cochlear implant survivors," who he said were "people who have been implanted and found that the device in fact was a failure, and have suffered as a result of the whole process." When I asked him how I could find out more about these "cochlear implant survivors," Gary suggested I contact Harlan Lane or the World Federation of the Deaf for stories of implant survivors. I later contacted both, but neither had any stories to share.

I did, however, locate a large-scale study by Cochlear Corporation,[25] of 5,300 users of the Nucleus implant device manufactured by the company. The study identified 174 non-users: people for whom the experience of getting an implant (although not necessarily the implant) was a failure. This group was divided into those who gave up their implant because of major surgical or medical problems (68), internal device failures (12), or unknown reasons (94). This gave an overall 3% non-use rate. Such a rate compares favorably with success rates for other surgical procedures on the ear, such as the replacement of middle ear bones.

Gary also talked about a study that showed that "73 percent of deaf children who have been implanted no longer use this device." I tracked this study down, and found that it was a survey of U.S. schools for the deaf.[26] The survey, undertaken by researchers at the Mayo Clinic in Jacksonville, Florida, had obtained replies from thirty (out of sixty-four) schools for the deaf, all of which were residential schools. Those schools reported having a combined total of seventy-five prelingually deaf children with cochlear implants, fifty-five of whom (73%) were no longer using the device. Residential schools for the deaf, however, are not the most congenial places for children to learn to hear and talk. The schools studied used a combination of sign language and speech called Total Communication, and such an environment may not provide a deaf child with the immersion in sound needed for successful rehabilitation (and habilitation).[27] The principal investigator for the study, Darrell Rose, took pains to point out that "these data may not reflect the same results for children in oral programs." In fact, about a third of all children in the United States with cochlear implants are in auditory/oral programs, and about a tenth or more are completely mainstreamed in regular schools.[28]

In the Cochlear Corporation study of 5,300 patients, non-use was most likely to happen in the case of adolescents. Twenty-one percent of prelingually deafened adolescents and 9% of postlingually deafened adolescents aged ten to seventeen had stopped using their implants at the time of the study. (Those deaf prelingually are those who were born profoundly deaf, or became profoundly deaf before they learned to speak.) Most researchers, and the adolescents themselves, attribute giving up the implant to peer pressure and concerns about appearance.[30]

Non-use for children in this same study was 4% for prelingually deaf children, and 2% for postlingually deaf children aged two to nine. These results may, however, understate the problem. For example, 20% of the prelingually and postlingually deaf children who consecutively received implants at the University of Iowa were reported in 1995 to have given up wearing their implants or be wearing them unreliably.[31] Even this figure, although sobering, was still nowhere near the 73% non-use figure in Rose's study.

Gary also claimed that there had been instances of fatalities caused by cochlear implants. A doctor in Austria had experimented

He didn't want to use his implant at all. He was struggling, trying to get by socially and academically, and he realized just how different he looked. The wires. The effort. He became angry and oppositional, talked back to teachers, got detentions.[29]

– Brent Sunderland, father of a fourteen-year-old who first received an implant at the age of two and stopped using it outside his home at the age of fourteen on deaf people, he said, and some patients had died. Yerker Andersson, the president of the World Federation of the Deaf, had heard the story from a social worker who knew the doctor. The social worker was now dead, and the doctor was unidentified. I told Gary that this was hearsay. There have been no cases anywhere of any death caused by a cochlear implant.[32] After trying to change my mind for a few moments, Gary reluctantly ceded my point, and I published the interview without this claim.

Gary Malkowski had suggested that I contact Professor Harlan Lane for information about "cochlear implant survivors." Lane is a specialist in the psychology of language and has written extensively on the subject of Deaf culture. A champion and spokesperson for the Deaf culture, he is himself hearing. Lane is opposed to cochlear implants in children and says that the devices would be wrong for children even if they worked perfectly.[33]

Lane had no stories of implant "survivors" for me. He sent me a pre-publication paper he had co-authored with Michael Grodin, the director of the Law, Medicine and Ethics Program at Boston University, entitled "Ethical Issues in Cochlear Implant Surgery: An Exploration into Disease, Disability, and the Best Interests of the Child." In that paper he and Grodin argue that hearing parents cannot be the best people to make a decision with respect to cochlear implants, because they cannot understand the culture to which their child "belongs" by virtue of the child's audiological deafness. As proof of this, the authors cite the fact that most Deaf adults do not want the procedure for themselves.[34] If the procedure is unwanted by mature members of the culture, according to Lane and Grodin's reasoning, it follows that the procedure is not in the best interest of a two-year-old deaf toddler with hearing parents either. This extrapolation, this proof, glosses over a lifetime of adaptation to deafness by Deaf people and glosses over the non-candidacy of most Deaf people for the procedure with a facileness that takes my breath away.

Parents who choose to get a cochlear implant for their child are often hurt by the accusation they are abusing their child for their own selfish reasons. On the CBS television program, "60 Minutes," Steven Parton, the father of Caitlin, who received an implant at the age of three, spoke eloquently for many of them. He said, "All we have done is given Caitie a tool and an option. She's experienced the delights of our culture that are not open to someone who cannot hear. That's not a small thing, to hear the spoken word and to hear the sounds of the world. And if Caitie chooses at some time in her life that these gifts are no longer pleasurable, she has the option to turn off the implant."[36]

> I want to have the implant. And – and I also – I wish I was like everyone else, you know. But I think I should have the implant. [35]
>
> – *Caitlin Parton, at the age of six*

The opposition to cochlear implants by the Deaf culture has a pervasive and perverse effect on children in residential schools for the deaf, and even on professionals working in the field. The Deaf children at residential schools for the deaf may absorb the opposition to implants and bully other children who have them. Unfortunately, this bullying and peer pressure may play a role in audiologists' decisions about candidacy, too. In one case that saddens me deeply, this opposition almost prevented a child who was becoming both deaf and blind from getting the little bit of sound that she wanted to help her cope with a world that was becoming increasingly devoid of both sound and sight.

Deborah Olk is the mother of two children with Usher's syndrome, a disease causing them to lose first their hearing and then their vision. Writing in the winter-spring 1995 issue of *CONTACT*, she recalled taking her daughters to Disney World. When they were leaving, she saw Jessica, her older daughter, signing to her little sister, "Remember everything you see. Because when we have to live in that dark and silent world, our memories will be all we have left."

When Jessica was sixteen, she decided she wanted a cochlear implant. Before her assessment at the clinic, the audiologist asked to meet with Jessica's mother. She was reluctant, the audiologist said, to approve Jessica for surgery. Jessica, she said, was too old to develop intelligible speech, but what is more important, she attended a residential school for the deaf. The audiologist and the clinic's implant surgeon had held an informal session on cochlear implants at Jessica's school several years ago and had been met by an angry student protest. The audiologist showed Deborah Olk pictures of the signs opposing cochlear implants that the students had carried. The audiologist felt that peer pressure would make Jessica uncomfortable with her implant, and most likely she would stop using it. Deborah Olk was appalled. All that she and Jessica hoped to get from an implant, she said, was an awareness of sound.

> Being deaf-blind is very lonely! ... It was obvious from the beginning that the CI would help to decrease my sense of isolation. I was now able to hear when a person came into my "space." I became aware of what was happening all around me. It's wonderful to have contact with reality. This may seem strange, but I also have more confidence in being in the dark now. [37]
>
> – Michelle Smithdas

Jessica's determination to hear, however, convinced the audiologist to go ahead with plans for the surgery. After Jessica's equipment was turned on, her mother took her to a store with music boxes from all over the world:

> The salesman took us to a beautiful wooden music box with a large gold wheel. He placed her hands on the box so she could feel what she was hearing. As Whitney Houston's "One Moment in Time" was playing, I explained to the salesman that Jessica had been deaf from birth and was hearing for the first time. I watched my daughter's face shine. Both of us cried tears of joy as she told me how beautiful the music was to her. It amazed her that there were little sounds inside of bigger sounds. Now she finally understood my love for music! As we walked back to the clinic, Jessica said, "Thank you, Mom, for the gift of hearing. I'm not afraid of that dark, silent world because it will be filled with sound."

Looking beyond the pathos of this story, the controversy over implanting children still has all the ingredients of a play by Becket with the characters not connecting and the tension never being resolved. Playing out their parts are the Deaf who see deafness as nothing to be fixed, the deaf who have cochlear implants and see deafness as a terrible and hated burden, and the medical professionals who see deafness as a deficit they can reduce. In the middle are caught the parents who need to make a choice and the children themselves who need to live with that choice. Confounding the issue are the facts that the children remain hearing impaired to varying degrees with their implant, and that it is difficult to predict how well they will do. Living with a hearing impairment will be a struggle no matter what choice their parents make.

> *I am twisted around in my eighth grade classroom seat, craning to see the boy at the back of the room who is responding to the teacher. I need to see his face so I can lipread. Everyone else, as usual, is sitting in straight rows, staring straight ahead. At me. One girl is doing more than that. She is grimacing and mouthing something to me. She says, "You're weird." I freeze. I cannot turn around and stare to the front like everyone else, even if that would make me un-weird. I cannot stay twisted around, watching the face of the boy, either. I am trapped in my weirdness.*

Ninety percent of children who are born deaf are born to families with hearing parents.[38] These parents may know nothing of deafness and are often devastated by the diagnosis of deafness. They may be bewildered and unsure of what steps to take to help their offspring. The Deaf culture and sign language may seem alien to them. They may want their child to be like them, to communicate in

The implant did not benefit me. It has been six years since my surgery and I never wear it. I think that hearing parents want the implant for their children because they want their children to be the same as them. What is wrong with being deaf?[39]

– Dawn Walker, aged seventeen, deafened at two and a half, received an implant at the age of eleven

the spoken language they use, and to share their values and pleasures in life. They may want their child to be able to freely communicate with everyone, not just those within the Deaf culture.

However, the studies of the efficacy of cochlear implants hold few definite promises. "The child," say experts in the field of pediatric implants, "will develop auditory skills gradually as a result of support and motivation."[40] The studies show that the procedure and devices have a low rate of failure, and typically provide the child with significant improvements in hearing over their pre-implant hearing level. Children, however, need to receive an implant soon after a diagnosis of deafness to reap the best advantage (although children receiving an implant later also benefit but more slowly), improvements take time, and the range of performance is very great, ranging from an ability to only better hear environmental sounds and to lipread with more ease, to being able to carry on interactive conversations over the phone with strangers. The bewildered parents may also be warned that the option of getting an implant will require the family to invest a great deal of time and resources in follow-up auditory therapy of some sort. The choice is not an easy one to make.

One person has likened having a disabled child to preparing for a trip to sunny Italy, buying all the right guidebooks and anticipating Michelangelo's David and the gondolas of Venice, then unexpectedly, landing in – Holland. There is disappointment, there may be grief, but there is also an opportunity to take pleasure in a new country, different from Italy, but still with its tulips and its Rembrandts, a beautiful country.[41]

Parents need to get as much information as possible about this new country and to make decisions based on their own family's circumstances.[43] They do not need to have a difficult situation made

> The battle is not over, but we are confident that David will achieve whatever he attempts. We still have to break ourselves from the habit of protecting him from everything. He still gets stared at and always will. All beautiful people do.[42]
>
> – Max Blum, father of David, who received a cochlear implant at two and a half

even more difficult by the addition of guilt and recrimination over their choice.

Deaf culture, like all cultures, represents an adaptation to a certain situation – in this case, deafness. And like all cultures, the Deaf culture has some wonderful attributes, many stemming from its own undeniably beautiful and rich language of signs. The Deaf can justifiably take pride in their culture and language, while acknowledging the history of oppression of deaf people. It would be tragic, however, if this newfound pride became the basis for yet another kind of oppression.

Cochlear implants are another adaptation to deafness. We who are deaf, whether we speak or sign or do both, share a very human ability to adapt and transform our lives according to our circumstances. I and other deaf adults should be able to choose freely the kind of adaptation we want to make, whether it be to get a cochlear implant or to adapt to deafness in other ways. And parents have a right, and even an obligation, to choose on behalf of their children what kind of adaptation they are prepared to support. It is true that none of the choices are easy, but they can and should be made with full information about the consequences, respect for those who choose differently, and without guilt for having rejected another's choice.

INTO THE FUTURE

Live as if everything is a miracle.
– Albert Einstein

Looking into the future, I expect that my deafness will become less and less of an inconvenience, even though I will remain deaf to some extent. Time and experience with my cochlear implant will help; so may new developments in implant technology and in biological remedies. I anticipate that the number of cochlear implant users will grow steadily, and the devices will become more widely available around the world. Perhaps one day, clinicians will also be better able to predict success with these devices, and scientists will narrow the confoundingly wide range of results so that more people are "high performers." In the meantime, I anticipate that deaf people will become increasingly proactive and will educate themselves about their options. We will also be helped by the informed social attitudes and the social support available to us that make it easier to be deaf today than it was when I was growing up.

The Americans with Disabilities Act has done much to heighten the awareness of North American society to the rights and needs of those with disabilities, and the media has been energetic in exploring the issues related to disabilities. There is no turning back. Ronald Reagan's hearing aid, and a former Miss America's[1] deafness

135

were both publicized extensively. The Deaf President Now movement was a proud moment in the history of U.S. Deaf culture, and with it came a fascination by the media with those who speak with their hands, and cannot hear. Some of this media exposure has benefitted oral deaf people too, although we are more hidden, integrated as we usually are in the hearing world. Our problems in living in a world where we are expected to hear remain less obvious.

I am at a meeting of a half-dozen organizations representing deaf and hard-of-hearing people. The guest speaker represents a coalition that intends to create an Ontarians with Disabilities Act much like the powerful Americans with Disabilities Act. He is blind and confesses that one of his fears in going on subways is of walking too far on the platform and falling over the edge, in front of an oncoming train. He tells us that this happens, and that a blind person in Toronto has been killed this way. I am horrified and ashamed that our society has been unable to free him of this terror. I think of my own private terror, which is of being shot by a policeman or robber who orders me, "Hands up," while I continue to walk or turn away from him unhearing. This does happen to deaf people: they are killed, due to a "misunderstanding."[2]

I can plug a jack into my processor directly from the stethoscope and hear everything, clear as a bell! Patients think I have a pretty high-tech stethoscope and I do! I carry a pager and can quickly respond by phone when needed. I'm even beginning to understand all the garble coming over the hospital loudspeakers. After just seven months with my CI, I feel my future is unlimited.[3]

– *Angelica Carranza, M.D., in 1994*

The greatest improvements with a cochlear implant are supposed to happen within the first six months or so of use. However, I continue to improve, and I do not think I have yet reached a plateau. While most people will gradually lose some of their hearing as they grow older, in my case, the reverse will be true. I am going to hear better as I age.

Dianne Allum-Mecklenburg and Gregorio Babighian, researchers writing from Germany and Italy respectively, have described how adult implant users who have been deaf for a long time improve more slowly and over a longer period than those deaf for a short period of time.[4] They found significant differences in the speech perception scores of adult implant users who had been deaf for a short time (less than three years) as opposed to those deaf for a long time (more than twenty years) – three years post-implant. But, amazingly, after more than five years of implant use, these differences between the two groups became insignificant. I have worn my implant system for barely five years, so I look forward to the possibility of even more improvements.

The authors, whose study is titled "Cochlear Implant Performance as an Indicator of Auditory Plasticity in Humans," say, "We are now at the point of being confident that learning-induced plasticity can be observed in deaf individuals of all ages who have received a cochlear implant." Based in part on their findings about improvements in adults after five years, the authors point out the potential for some deaf children who receive their implants at a later age to do well, and possibly, with time, catch up to some extent with children implanted earlier. Time can be a great leveler.

In the same paper, Drs. Mecklenburg and Babighian mention in passing how we might promote improvements, encouraging the natural plasticity of our auditory systems. They tantalizingly suggest that in the future this might be through the use of electrical signals from more advanced technologies, pharmaceutical treatment or possibly a combination of the two. In the case of advanced technologies, they point to increasingly sophisticated device processing strategies that are being developed; in the case of pharmaceutical treatment, they say that treatment with neural growth factors or neurotransmitters may facilitate change.

We already know that electrical stimulation in animals can partially prevent and reverse the degeneration of the auditory system following deafness.[5] Neuroscientists around the world are also working on the problem of how to chemically activate healing and growth in damaged neural tissue. These treatments would be useful in cases such as spinal cord injuries, Parkinson's disease, and other disorders. Scientists have identified a whole family of nerve growth factors, some of which promote neural survival (and possibly plasticity) in different animals, in different parts of their bodies. The trick is to identify the appropriate ones for specific parts of the body and determine if they can safely regenerate neuronal systems without adversely affecting other parts of the body. If scientists identify such a chemical, which promotes central auditory system plasticity (in the brain), then in the future, they might be able to treat sensorineural deafness like mine by means of an injection of drugs, either alone or in combination with a cochlear implant.

Scientists are also working in several centers around the world to determine how to specifically regenerate inner-ear hair cells. The hair cells of the inner ear are crucial in conveying sound information from the ear to the auditory nerve, and typically, they are damaged in cases of severe and profound deafness. Edwin Rubel and Brenda Ryals were among the first scientists to discover the possibility of ear hair cell regeneration in birds.[6] They found that after birds' inner-ear hair cells had been destroyed by noise or drugs in the laboratory, the birds became deaf, but within days, they grew new inner-ear hair cells that almost completely restored their hearing. This was a revolutionary finding, since everyone previously believed that once these hair cells were destroyed, permanent deafness was inevitable. Looking at how well cochlear implant users can do with just a few channels of electrical information replacing 15,000 ear hair cells, Dr. Rubel says he is excited about what the regeneration of just a hundred or so of these hair cells might do.[7] So am I.

But will I and others with cochlear implants be eligible for this treatment in the future? Will those with cochlear implants be shut out from taking advantage of these developments because of damage done to their ears by the insertion of an electrode array? When I asked Dr. Rubel in 1997 if implanting my other ear might limit my ability to make use of ear hair cell regeneration should that become a reality, he cautioned me that it might:

Research on hair cell regeneration is very early. The findings that this was possible in birds were only ten years
ago, and it wasn't until the last couple of years that we
have [begun] experimentally trying to induce such abili-
ties in mammals. Thus it is way too early to attempt an
accurate prediction of when it may be possible to induce
this remarkable feat in humans. I do believe that long
term insertion of a cochlear implant will do damage to
the cells that might potentially be the source of regenerated hair cells. In addition, mechanical properties of the
inner ear would likely be disrupted by insertion or
removal of a cochlear implant. Thus, implanting a second ear would probably prevent regeneration and/or prevent the regenerated hair cells from being appropriately
stimulated by sound. This is an opinion, and before a
definitive answer is given, animal experiments would be
required.[8]

Dr. Ryals answers the question of when human ear hair cell
regeneration might be feasible by saying that it "may be as close as
tomorrow in humans, or it may never be possible."[9] Dr. Ryals also
points out that finding a way to stimulate hair cell regeneration in
humans is only a beginning. Some deaf people might not be candidates because of a pathological condition of their inner ear. She cau-
tions that at this point we do not know if early efforts at hair cell
regeneration will be an improvement over the benefit provided by
cochlear implants. There are simply more unknowns when it comes
to hair cell regeneration in the inner ear than there are for cochlear
implants.

If I should, however, leave one ear free for future developments,
this presents a dilemma both for me and others who may wish to
upgrade their current implant. Most surgeons (including my own)
are reluctant to remove a functioning device and replace it with
another that *might* be better (or might not). As one surgeon who I
consulted said, there is a danger that in doing so, he might inflict

harm (contrary to the Hippocratic oath), because the second implant might not work as well as the first. There are never any guarantees with cochlear implant (or any other) surgery. So some surgeons would opt to implant the other ear. This, of course, would leave no ear free of implantation and available for developments such as ear hair cell regeneration. I've thought often that I really need three ears.

Moreover, even if a surgeon were prepared to replace an implant in the same ear, he or she could encounter problems if the new electrode array were thicker or longer than the old. Surgeons have told me that after an electrode array has been inside the ear for a long time, it normally becomes encased in a fibrous sheath. They can slip an electrode array out of its fibrous sheath and surgically insert a new one of the same size or smaller, usually with little problem. It may, however, be difficult for them to insert a new one of a larger size without trauma to the ear. The issue of implant upgrades is not a simple one.

Upgrades are going to become more of a concern to implant users in the future when newer multichannel devices provide a clear benefit over older ones (some would say that day is fast approaching, or may even be here). Implant users and clinicians will also want to know more about how two implants can coexist. After all, hearing people benefit from hearing with two ears: they can better determine where a sound is coming from, and they can hear better in ambient noise with two ears than with one. So far, however, there have been few cases of people with multichannel implants in both ears, although some people with older single-channel implants have had those implants removed and replaced with a newer multichannel implant. As well, some people have left their single-channel implant in one ear and received a newer implant in the other. But there have not been many cases of people with two functioning multichannel implants. The benefit of two (binaural) cochlear implants has not really been demonstrated.[10] Sometimes, where two multichannel implants coexist, the wearer turns one implant off or finds that wearing two does not really give much benefit. Once more people seek and obtain a second implant, however, we may learn more about this type of fitting. Some researchers believe that two implants may be more effective together if both are of the same type, which further complicates the whole issue of upgrading implants for those who have an older one.[11]

I fully expect to get a second cochlear implant someday. If it would help me to hear better, I would welcome an upgrade even if it involved a second surgery. I wouldn't even mind a period during which I needed to become accustomed to a new set of sounds. (I have kept my audiotape of Make Way for Ducklings at the ready.) I wear my old hearing aid in my non-implanted ear occasionally (when I remember to put it in) on the chance that it will help to keep that ear alive for a second implant.[12] I don't seem to hear much with it and don't even realize sometimes when its battery has run down. However, it makes everything seem a bit louder, even in my implanted ear, and when I wear it, it seems like I am hearing from the middle of my head rather than from one side.

It appears I am unusual in welcoming the idea of a second implant. In talking to others, I find that most people would not opt for a second surgery, even if they could persuade their insurance company or government agency to fund it (and this could be a problem except in cases of clear failure of the older implant).

Most people seem content with what they have: surveys show that cochlear implant users have a very high level of satisfaction. One of the first such reports of subjective benefit, a 1994 report from my own clinic in Toronto, analyzed responses from twenty of twenty-three consecutively implanted postlingually deaf adult implant users, and seventeen of their relatives.[13] The clinic found that 85% of the patients and 94% of their relatives were moderately to very satisfied with their device. The implant users said they had experienced substantial improvements in speech recognition with lipreading, in voice quality, independence, and communication confidence.

More recently (in 1997), a researcher in Australia reported on the psycho-social benefit of cochlear implants for 129 adults.[14] He found that they felt significantly less anxious and more confident about social interaction and about their future than deaf adults without implants. His qualitative analysis of interview data is a good testimonial to the benefits of hearing with a cochlear implant: "Implantation meant that they felt connected to the world. ... Partners were less stressed by everyday communication while spontaneous family interactions and social outings increased. ... It meant not being afraid of talking to strangers; being able to talk to people at the bus stop; no longer being afraid of meeting and talking to people at the local shops or bank."

The meetings I attend of my local cochlear implant support group are like old-fashioned religious revival meetings. People have what I call a "post-implant zest." They stand up to introduce themselves, with eyes shining, saying, "I got my implant on May 23, 1994, and it's a miracle!" And: "I got mine in February 1997, and it's changed my life." And: "I received my implant on December 15, 1996, and this gift of hearing was the best Christmas present I ever got!" I find the testimonials both hokey and touching.

There were more testimonials to the miraculous nature of cochlear implants at the Cochlear Implant Club International convention in 1997, which attracted an astounding 800 attendees to Sturbridge, Massachusetts. Warm feelings and camaraderie flowed freely. I cannot imagine a group of hearing-aid users coming together from around the world in a comparable emotion-charged event. At one session, offered by an implant manufacturer, a man in the audience got up to scold the company's representative for not paying enough attention to those with older implants that cannot run some of the newer processing strategies. But after he sat down, others in

> Max began hearing in May. He had a big spoken vocabulary of nouns, adjectives, and verbs by September and he began using sentences in December (usually to turn his nose up at foods he does not like: "C'est pas bon, ça!"). ... Max seems to love his implant. He gets up most mornings and asks for it. He once gave it a kiss.[15]
>
> – *Celeste Coleon, Paris, France, mother of three-year-old Max, who received his implant in May 1996*

the audience stood up to insist that they were happy with what they had, that they had no desire for anything more than what they were getting, that what they had was a "miracle."

When I first started investigating a multichannel cochlear implant in 1992, there were only about 7,000 people around the world who wore the devices. Today, there are around 20,000[16] in more than seventy countries. In the United States, approximately 10% of all profoundly deaf children from newborn to eighteen had a cochlear implant as at July 1, 1994.[17] One device manufacturer projects that by the year 2002, there will be 45,000 users, world-wide.[18] Moreover, a second company predicts that by that same year, children will outnumber adults as new users, with up to 70% of new cochlear implant recipients being children.[19]

These figures, however, barely address the large numbers of deaf and severely hard-of-hearing people who could benefit from a cochlear implant. One manufacturer estimates that each year, 20,000 new cases of profound hearing loss and 52,000 cases of severe hearing loss occur that are eligible for cochlear implantation in the company's core markets, which include Australia, the United States, Western European countries, and Japan.[20] But only a small portion of these people go on to get the device. A huge gap exists between eligibility for and actual receipt of a cochlear implant.

This gap occurs for many reasons. First of all, not enough people are familiar with cochlear implants and what they can do. Family doctors, for example, may not refer eligible deaf people to implant clinics, because the doctors may be unaware of the procedure or may not understand the eligibility criteria or benefits that cochlear implants can bring. Second, many deaf people and parents of deaf children may be reluctant to proceed because of a fear of the surgery that is often fed by media reports that erroneously call it "brain surgery." Third, not all otolaryngologists or hospitals are able to perform this specialized surgery, and there is a relative scarcity of implant clinics. And finally, and perhaps of most importance, there is insufficient funding. Even in the United States, with its mix of

Medicare and private health insurance, cochlear implant surgeon Noel Cohen, of the New York University Medical Center, says that his major problem today as an implant surgeon is – funding.

Where the main source of funding is private insurance companies, as in the United States, some companies refuse to pay for cochlear implants, wrongly believing they are just updated versions of a hearing aid.[21] In countries where the source of funding is the government, as it is in Canada and the United Kingdom, allocations are rarely sufficient. Indeed, at the Fifth International Cochlear Implant Conference in New York City in 1997, presenters from Latin America, England, and the United States (as well as individuals I spoke to from Australia and Canada) noted that a major problem they repeatedly encounter is the lack of adequate funding. Sue Archbold of Nottingham, England, said that her program's major problem in the past, present, and future was "funding, funding, and funding."[22]

At least three developments in implant technology will likely encourage the wider use of cochlear implants and change the ways in which they are worn: behind-the-ear processors, combination hearing aids and processors, and auditory brainstem implants.

In 1997, one of the multichannel device manufacturers introduced a behind-the-ear processor that looks much like a regular behind-the-ear hearing aid (but with a thin cable linking it to a transmitter coil resting on the scalp). This is an important milestone in the development of cochlear implants and will likely culminate in a few years in a completely implantable processor that will be externally invisible. I no longer find my equipment bulky or particularly inconvenient, although I would find a behind-the-ear processor more comfortable to wear. I have become accustomed to my equipment and would never count it as a major consideration in light of the benefit my implant system brings. If it would help me to hear better, I would gladly carry around something much bigger and heavier than I do now. In spite of increased acceptance of deafness, however, many people, especially teenagers, resist wearing a device that draws attention to their deafness. It is possible that deaf people and parents of deaf children who recoil from the seemingly awkward equipment of some implant systems will look more favorably on this device and procedure, if they can obtain good benefit with a less obtrusive device. This development may help to swell the numbers of implant users.

Another development in progress is the use of the devices with hearing aids. With more adults who have significant residual hearing (i.e., those who are severely hearing-impaired rather than profoundly deaf) becoming eligible for the procedure, the use of hearing aids with implants is receiving more attention from researchers and clinicians. Many people with a severe hearing impairment can still use hearing aids with some benefit. Work is underway in Australia on a "combionic" aid that combines the signal of a cochlear implant processor and a hearing aid in one unit.[23]

A third development that may expand the numbers of users involves the auditory brainstem implant (ABI). This device, which works like a cochlear implant but bypasses the ear completely, is still in its infancy. Its use will likely grow for those who cannot benefit from a cochlear implant. More people may become eligible for it: not only those with neurofibromatosis as is the case now, but also those who have been considered ineligible for a cochlear implant because of inner ear malformations. We no longer need an ear with which to hear.

The criteria for cochlear implant eligibility have become less restrictive as results have improved. And results have improved not only because of advances in the technology, but also because of the

> I am perversely proud that ... I learnt sign language about the same time I received my precious implant. I'm active in both the Brisbane [Australia] cochlear implant group and the Deaf community – two very different worlds. ... Occasionally I can correct some of the misconceptions about the implant still prevalent within the Deaf community ("Yes I have a shower every day").[24]
>
> – Nancy Hoffmann, who received an implant forty-one years after becoming profoundly deaf from meningitis at the age of six

greater experience of the clinical professionals and better selection of appropriate candidates. I am optimistic that with more careful selection of candidates, improved support for implant users, and more information about the safety and efficacy of cochlear implants and the joy they can bring to both children and adults, people in the Deaf culture will be less likely to oppose the procedure. I hope too that this book will build a bridge to the Deaf culture and help to remove some of the misunderstandings upon which much of the opposition is based.

In the last stages of writing this book, I received a fax from a woman I had contacted for permission to quote from a letter she had written to a magazine. The letter was a cry from the heart, telling how she had been coaxed into getting an implant at the age of fifteen, with visions of hearing dangled in front of her eyes. She had become deaf from meningitis at the age of five and had been mainstreamed in her local school. She came from a small town and had been one of the first children to have the procedure at the city hospital she went to. She said her cochlear implant had been a failure, and after she got it she entered one of the darkest periods of her life. I wanted to excerpt her letter in my book, to include her voice. I hoped to show that not everyone finds cochlear implants miraculous devices, that it doesn't work out for everyone. It seemed, when I read her letter, that she was an example of a poor candidate – she had not wanted the procedure to start with, and she had been given an implant at a difficult time – her teen years. Teenagers understandably don't have the maturity to deal with the challenge of hearing differently, and being different, and they don't have the pliability of a child.

When I called her on my TTY, she readily agreed to give me permission to quote from her letter. I told her a bit about my book, and about how I wanted to present as many views as possible, to show the wide range of responses that people have both to cochlear implants and to deafness itself. I went on to say that I would like her to understand that I wear a cochlear implant myself, and that my experience with it has been relatively successful. She tried to explain to me why hers was not. She said that when she got it, everything was loud and strange. She did not like the sounds and could not make sense of them so she stopped using it.

I did not get a chance to ask her how long she tried for, but it was probably irrelevant. If she had no mentor, no support in her small town, knew no other people with implants, then what were her chances at the age of fifteen, several years ago, of succeeding with this device? I told her that I wished her well, and then I had to hang up as there was someone at the door.

Later, she wrote me an impassioned, articulate fax. After thinking it over, she said, she had changed her mind; she was annoyed that I had made a point of telling her how my own implant had been successful. It seemed to her that I had been trying to compare myself with her and to underline her failure. She did not want to be named in my book as an example of a cochlear implant failure because she feared I would use her story as ammunition against the Deaf culture and deaf children. I felt anguished, and as if I had been kicked in the stomach. I had told her about myself simply to put the facts on the table and be fair to her so she would know I was not a member of the Deaf culture, and I was not about to write an anti-cochlear implant book. She could not, after all, see me, or hear my tone of voice because we were talking over the TTY. And my motives in using her quotation were the opposite of what she thought. Rather than as ammunition against the Deaf culture, her quotation was to help readers of this book understand that the experience of getting an implant is not always a happy one, that some people may not be good candidates, and that their experience in getting an implant can be very painful.

We cannot expect to eradicate deafness in the foreseeable future. As Dr. Noel Cohen says, some people will not want to have their hearing "fixed," and in any case we are not wise enough to remedy all cases of deafness.[25] The World Health Organization estimates that more than 80% of the world's 120 million people with disabling hearing difficulties live in developing countries.[26] Moreover, because of intermarriage (which promotes genetic problems), poor hygiene (which promotes infections), and poor training of medical practitioners, hearing loss is more prevalent in developing countries than in those that are more developed. For example, in China, a primary cause of hearing loss, especially in children, is the improper administration of antibiotics such as neomycin and kanamycin by the "barefoot doctors" who received no formal medical training during the Cultural Revolution of the 1960s and 1970s.

> We believe that there are powers beyond our control, beyond anyone's control, and that Deaf people are in this world for mysterious and unknown reasons. Brenda [Mowl's wife] and I, therefore, ... cannot and will not support the genetic engineering research and development that will lead to a perfect race nor will we use the option of cochlear implants for our children.[28]
>
> — Gary E. Mowl, who has three children with a hearing loss and comes from a family that has been Deaf and hard of hearing for four generations

For those living in developing countries, however, the $20,000 U.S. price of cochlear implant equipment (in 1998) is prohibitive[27], and the expertise for the surgery and follow-up care may be scarce. This situation may change in the future: work is underway at the House Ear Institute in Los Angeles to develop a low-cost cochlear implant that could be used in developing countries.

One of the reasons why cochlear implants are so intriguing is that they show how little we understand about the brain and the mystery of how we hear. We do not completely understand the intricate pathways that sound takes from the ear to the comprehending brain, nor how language, that most complex of sound information, is processed. And because these are mysteries still, the future for cochlear implants is all the more exciting.

For now, cochlear implants are, as one scientist says, a great "trick of the mind." Sending just a few channels of electrical information to replace the functioning of approximately 15,000 ear hair cells in the normal ear, cochlear implants trick the mind into believing it is hearing symphonies, speech, and birdsong.

The challenge is to harness this "trick" to ensure that everyone does well with his or her implant system. Clinicians cannot accurately predict how well people will do with their implant before they get one. Because they still cannot fully explain why some people do so much better than others, they are unable to help some people make better use of their implants.

Perhaps the biggest challenge that lies ahead is not to make the devices smaller and more cosmetically appealing but to narrow the wide range of performance, so that everyone or almost everyone becomes a "high performer."

In the early days, researchers thought that many electrodes and channels of information (i.e., pairs of electrodes between which current flows) would be needed to approximate normal hearing with an implant. However, Dr. Robert Shannon, director of Auditory Implant Research at the House Ear Institute, and his colleagues have done experiments with current devices that show that in experimental conditions when some functioning electrodes are turned off, people can hear just as well with a few electrodes delivering a few channels of information as with many electrodes delivering more channels of information (within limits).[30] They say that this just underlines how little we still understand about how patients make use of the electrical signals their implants provide.

Dr. Shannon, in 1996, published a wonderful article free of jargon and waffling in the journal *Seminars in Hearing*. It is called "Cochlear Implants: What Have We Learned and Where Are We Going."[31] In it, he claims that we may have reached a point of overkill in the technology of cochlear implants, that we can provide many channels of less than optimum information, but haven't yet figured out how to adjust the fitting for a patient to deliver just a few

> No one really understands this truly incredible ability we possess that enables us to distinguish speech and environmental sounds with vastly less information than the normal hearing ear receives. I believe it is our faith in this unknown potential that allows us to bond to the implant, to make its sounds a familiar part of us.[29]
>
> – *cochlear implant user Larry Orloff*

channels of information optimally. He warns that because we do not understand why the devices work as well as they do, we are in danger of running out of one of the key factors that has led to our success to date: "serendipity."

Dr. Shannon suggests that much of the variability in how well patients do may stem from the fact that they are not fitted appropriately with their devices, and we do not yet know enough about how to custom-fit devices for each patient. Many audiologists with whom I have spoken agree with Dr. Shannon. They say their fittings of patients are often by trial and error, and they would benefit from more guidelines for what should be tried with certain patients. In addition, they would like to be able to prescribe one device as opposed to another for a certain patient because that device is a better fit. Much more research is needed, however, before they can do so.

In the meantime, candidates will continue to be told that their performance cannot be accurately predicted. They may also be told that there are no reliably significant differences in performance capability between currently available devices, and that they need to decide which device they want based on other factors such as the attributes of the external equipment or the device manufacturers, or which device they can more easily get reimbursed for. Today, because the technology is continuously changing, device comparisons are especially difficult to make. If two devices are compared at one point in time, by the time information about differences in performance emerges, the device that fared worse may have been upgraded. And so a new round of comparisons would be needed. Some candidates will throw up their hands and ask their surgeon to decide which implant they should get. After receiving their implant, many will patiently sit in front of their audiologist during their periodic tuning sessions and simply conform to the standard procedures the audiologist uses in setting their comfort levels and thresholds. Most audiologists have a very limited amount of time to experiment with different fittings, although most do their best.

Believing that little can be done to help them hear even better, some deaf people may not ask for any specific adjustments in their processor's program and will pose few questions for their audiologist. For example, one adult I know used to turn off her processor each time she flushed a toilet. The sound was so loud and harsh she could not bear it. Then she heard about others who asked their audiologists to adjust their processors for uncomfortable sounds. She worked up the nerve to do the same, her audiologist made a simple adjustment, and she was finally able to flush a toilet without switching her processor off.

There are many ways in which deaf people can be proactive in obtaining the best benefit of cochlear implant technology. It may not be everyone's way; moreover, being proactive does not guarantee we will do better with our cochlear implants. But we may find the feeling of involvement satisfying.

We can educate ourselves about this technology. We can join one of the Internet discussion groups to talk to others with implants, extending our community to encompass the world. We can do searches of the literature on MEDLINE in order to navigate our way around the capabilities of the various devices (see the Resources section at the back of this book). We can research the merits of different implant brands, review performance studies, and investigate manufacturers' plans for the future. We can join a local support group if there is one (or form one if there isn't), and talk to other implant users about their satisfaction with their devices. We can read journals and newsletters with articles about cochlear implants. We can question the experience of surgeons and audiologists performing implantation, seeking out those professionals who have more experience. We can also determine the follow-up rehabilitation programs that are available at the different clinics. Then, having completed our research, we can decide on a device and clinic accordingly, although for many of us, the decision will be constrained by where we live and restrictions on the funding available to us.

After we get our implants, we can participate in research studies through our clinics. These studies will be important in helping the technology and the clinical practice to advance. When we go into our clinic for device fittings, we may be prepared with knowledge and understanding obtained from our research and from talking to other users. We can discuss various options with our audiologists (learning more in the process), and together with our audiologists experiment with different device settings. We can ask about patch cords that allow us to hook our processors up directly to a Walkman, or about FM or infrared devices we can use with our implant systems at movie theaters and lectures. My own hard-working audiologist has probably come to expect the point in our sessions when I reach into my purse to bring out my list of questions and things for us to try together in my never-ending quest for better hearing.

Our options are many, our resources for evaluating them are rich, and we are situated at a point in history where we can influence the options available to those who follow us. It is as a partner that I go into the future with other deaf people, and with the audiologists, surgeons, and scientists who are developing this technology that can transform the lives of deaf people.

EPILOGUE

It has now been five years since that hot, loud day when my cochlear implant was first turned on. The beeps and buzzes that I heard then now seem like normal hearing. I feel sometimes as if I have always heard this way, as if I always knew what the letter *s* sounded like, that plastic bags make a rustling sound, and that a pencil makes a scratching noise when I write with it on a piece of paper. I still discover new sounds, however, realizing what I have missed. Just last month, walking within my house, I stopped and listened: for the first time, I heard the sound of rain on my roof. And words and sentences still waft toward me, for me to pluck them out of the air and understand them where before I would not even have known that they had been spoken.

When I struggle with a difficult voice on the phone or cannot understand a news announcer with a deep bass voice on the radio, I feel a twinge of regret that I do not hear even better than I am hearing now and an annoyance that I am still deaf. But then I chastise myself for my greediness, remembering that before I got my implant, I would not have understood anyone at all on the phone, and the radio would have been just noise. And in a small corner of my mind, I will hope to do even better, resolving to take this technology as far as it will go.

My cochlear implant has given me a rear-view mirror onto my deafness. It illuminates, often in a startlingly harsh light, what I have missed in being deaf since childhood, and allows me to see what I adapted to as I grew into deafness. The joy with which deaf people like myself greet the sounds given to us by our cochlear implants highlights the loss and emptiness so many of us feel as a result of a world gone silent.

Am I "out" of deafness? Yes, and no. When I talk to another person or a few people, in a quiet spot, I feel that I have come out of deafness, and that I am deaf no more. I no longer strain, intent on

153

catching every movement of the other person's lips: I hear with ease. When I speak to people on the telephone and have a long conversation with them, asking that they repeat just a few words or phrases, I thrill to my new skill and feel I have come out of deafness to a state where I am merely hard of hearing, not deaf. But, then, I will find myself with too many people talking all at once, in a place where there is too much noise, and I will feel once again very deaf. I will be back inside my old deafness. And, when my battery runs down or I am swimming in the lake without my external hearing equipment, I hear absolutely nothing. I am deaf.

In many ways, however, I do feel "out." Although I grew up ashamed of my deafness, unable to reveal myself as deaf to others, preferring even to be considered foolish (foolish enough to not even be able to point out the equator on a map), I no longer feel this way. Rather than feel shame for my deafness, I now know I have much to be proud of, in having coped with such a huge disability. Social attitudes toward disabilities have changed, and so have I. Even as my deafness has become much less disabling, I have come far in understanding it and acknowledging what I previously hid or bluffed away. It is as if this technology deep within my ear has brought my little secret of deafness out in the open, and it has empowered and emboldened me.

There is much that I have learned on this journey through deafness. I have a new respect for how I and other deaf people are able to "hear" with what little hearing we may have (with and without a cochlear implant); I have a new appreciation for the delights of sounds now that I can hear so many of them. This fresh understanding has given me a new sense of fellowship with other deaf people, although I grew up knowing none other than my father. I also feel fortunate in having gained a feeling of partnership with science and technology that I did not have before, when I was sitting at the sidelines, waiting for the miraculous to happen.

Reading my story of growing into deafness and learning about the price I paid for living as if I were a hearing person in a hearing milieu, without sign language, with few accommodations, and little acceptance of my deafness, some will say that I would have been better off growing up within the Deaf culture. There, I could have communicated with my hands and body by signing (with those who knew how to sign). There, I could have found acceptance and never be called "weird" (at least while I was with members of the Deaf culture). I would not have had to struggle to be something I was not. It is true that it would have been better if I had been able to acknowledge and accept my deafness rather than try to pass as hearing, and I realize that I have paid a high price for growing up as I did. Being where I am now, however, it is not possible for me or anyone else to fairly judge whether I would have been better off growing up within the embrace of the signing Deaf community.

Although hearing people are now more aware of those in the Deaf culture, and more ready to accommodate them with both acceptance and sign language interpreters, nonetheless, the signing Deaf are still limited by the simple fact that most people do not sign. I am therefore thankful for the wider world that I have been part of for having grown up "oral deaf," the broad education I have received, the wide variety of hearing friends I have, the opportunities that would not have been mine were I part of the Deaf culture. Moreover, if I had been part of that culture, it is unlikely that I would have been able to taste the sweet pleasure of traveling out of deafness and into more hearing, with my cochlear implant. To those who would argue that the price has been too high, I say no, it has been worth it.

My cochlear implant has made my life much easier, but it has not made me hearing. I am still hearing-impaired, and my life is more complicated for that reason. For example, a little while ago, I attended a conference in New York City. I was unable to simply reserve a hotel room, book a flight, and register for the conference. I needed to request in advance that the hotel provide me with a flashing strobe alert system that would wake me if there was a fire while I was asleep with my processor turned off and lying useless on the table beside my bed. When I boarded my plane, I had to explain to the flight stewardess that I would not understand any of the announcements blared out over the public address system. I asked her to come to my seat to tell me of any important ones. If there was a problem, and we were diverted to another airport, for example, I wanted to know about it in advance, not when I stumbled off the plane. And, at the conference itself, I needed to ask the organizers to provide me with an assistive listening system (FM or infrared) that I could plug into my processor, so I would not be listening to speeches all day without comprehending them. These devices can be wonderful in bringing the speaker's voice clearly and directly to my processor, as if the speaker were only inches away from me.

When I finally took my place in the audience, I was dismayed to find that the auditorium was darkened, and I would be unable to lipread the speakers. I started to feel my old panicky feelings of helplessness. Then I plugged myself in to the FM system that had been provided to me, tuned in, and surprised even myself by understanding, for most of the talks, all or almost all that was said. I felt myself swell with pride.

If there is one message that I would give to parents of deaf children it is that they acknowledge and accept their child's deafness, and help their child to do the same. No deaf child should be encouraged to "pass" as hearing, nor feel ashamed of being deaf. Parents who choose a cochlear implant for their deaf child are facing their child's disability head-on, rather than trying to hide it. The visibility of the current devices prevents that, but also the rehabilitation with therapists and teachers and audiologists that most children obtain following their surgery empowers them, giving them a wide network of support from caring adults in dealing with their deafness. I wish I had had that kind of support growing up deaf.

Discoveries of deafness in a child, like my own when a nail clipping flew into my eye and my family realized my need to lipread, will continue to be traumatic for many hearing families. Learning that their child is deaf will probably always be painful for them.

They may feel a loss, and grieve for what could have been. But as David Luterman reminds us:

> Happiness, say the poets, is a matter of having something to do, someone to love, and something to hope for. Deafness gives you all of this in full measure. At the very least, this [deaf] child has ensured that you will have a very interesting life.[1]

There are few medical procedures for which patients need one another more than they do for cochlear implantation. We need not only improved technology and improved device fittings, but also we need each other. Those of us who are deaf can learn from each other what the hearing professionals cannot understand, cannot explain, and cannot advise us on, in spite of their dedication and knowledge. We can share with one another and with those who are hearing, the experience of deafness, and the experience of hearing with this new technology. My understanding of my own deafness still unfolds, and the folds cannot be turned back and pressed shut on deafness.

Wings across the blue
The only way out is through[2]

ENDNOTES

PROLOGUE

1. The Canadian Hearing Society, *Hearing Loss: Questions and Answers*, May 1991, p. 2.

2. M. Leske, "Prevalence Estimates of Communicative Disorders in the U.S.," *ASHA* 23 (1981): 229-327 as cited in J.G. Kyle et al., "Adjustment to Acquired Hearing Loss: A Working Model," in *Adjustment to Adult Hearing Loss*, ed. H. Orlans (San Diego: College-Hill Press, 1985), p. 119.

3. The Listening Center at Johns Hopkins, *Bringing Sound to Life for Deaf Children* (brochure).

4. The Canadian Hearing Society, *Hearing Loss: Questions and Answers*, May 1991, p. 2; Canadian Hearing Society Bulletin CHS94102-05. The number of deaf persons in the United States, however, has been revised downward by the National Institute on Deafness and Other Communication Disorders (NIDCD) from 2 million "profoundly deaf" in 1988, to 421,000 who are "deaf in both ears" in 1994 (.18% of the population). The difference in the numbers reveals how statistics can be greatly affected by definitions of who is "deaf"; moreover, self-identification of the deaf in surveys can be unreliable. For estimates, see the current "NIDCD Fact Sheet: Statistics on Deafness and Hearing Disorders in the United States."

CHAPTER 1

1. Helen Keller, *The Story of My Life* (Garden City, New York: Doubleday, 1954), p. 374. Keller was deaf and blind from the age of nineteen months.

2. Dianne Allum-Mecklenburg, presentation at Cochlear Implant Club International Convention, Sturbridge, Massachusetts, 1997.

3. An implant system is under development in 1998 to make use

of the middle ear's conductive properties. A. Zhang et al., "The Development of a Tympanic Membrane Sensor for a Totally Implantable Cochlear Implant or Hearing Aid" in *Cochlear Implants: XVI World Congress of Otorhinolaryngology Head and Neck Surgery, Sydney (Australia), 1997*, ed. G.M. Clark (Bologna: Monduzzi Editore, 1996).

4. Kristin A. Buehl, from a message posted on the Internet CI Forum, September 28, 1997. Used with permission.

5. Douglas P. Lynch, Cochlear Implant Users' Panel, Self-Help for Hard of Hearing (SHHH) Convention, Phoenix, Arizona, June 1997.

6. Angela Theriault as quoted in Dale Anne Freed, "Deaf Protest Use of Hearing Device," *The Toronto Star*, May 14, 1994, p. A4.

7. Gil McDougald, "Hearing the Crowd Roar Again," 1995 Cochlear Implant Club International Keynote Speech, *CONTACT*, Fall 1995, p. 17.

8. "A Mildly Luddite Love Song," Copyright Howard L. Kaplan. Used with permission.

9. I had some tinnitus before getting my implant, and although I did experience some in the few days after my turn on, it eventually decreased and virtually disappeared (manifesting only occasionally and only when I am without my processor turned on). Generally, cochlear implantation has a beneficial effect on tinnitus. For example, in one study, 46 of 110 patients showed a significant improvement in their tinnitus following implantation (J.W.P. Hazell et al., "Mechanisms of Tinnitus in Profound Deafness," *Proceedings of the International Cochlear Implant Speech and Hearing Symposium* [Melbourne, 1994], p. 418). However, increased tinnitus is a possible negative outcome of implantation and was observed in 15 of 3,064 adults in another study. Eleven of the fifteen patients experienced permanent increased tinnitus. For the other four, the increase was transient, as it was in my case. (R. A. Hoffman, N.L. Cohen, "Complications of Cochlear Implant Surgery," *Proceedings of the International Cochlear Implant Speech and Hearing Symposium* [Melbourne, 1994], p. 420.)

10. Kay Basham, "Love, Laughter, and Music," *CONTACT*, Summer 1993, p. 10.

11. Under controlled situations, with a well-secured implant, even those with implanted magnets as part of their cochlear implant systems may be able to undergo MRI, according to reports at the Fifth International Cochlear Implant Conference in New York, 1997 (W. Baumgartner et al., "Magnetic Resonance Imaging in Cochlear Implanted Patients"; C.H. Chouard et al., "Magnetic Resonance Imaging and Cochlear Implants"; C. Teissl et al., "Magnetic Resonance Imaging Compatibility of a Cochlear Implant"). Some newer devices also allow a surgeon to remove the magnet from the implant and then replace it after the MRI is complete.

12. Cathy Este (Simon), as quoted in June Epstein, *The Story of the Bionic Ear* (Melbourne: Hyland House, 1989), p. 127.

CHAPTER 2

1. "What You Do With What You've Got," Si Kahn, Joe Hill Music (ASCAP). Used with permission.

2. Meri Garst, "A Bionic Hearing Aid," *CONTACT*, Winter/Spring 1997, p. 20.

3. A. Boothroyd et al., "Responses of Cochlear Implantees to Speech Perception Training," presentation to Annual Convention of American Speech, Language and Hearing Association, New Orleans, 1987.

4. When I later contacted Arthur Boothroyd, he said that his 1987 study, although it was interpreted by many to mean that rehabilitation was not needed, also showed that the key to the more successful subjects was a combination of an effective implant, and the confidence and willingness to engage in spoken language communication ("time on task"): "What I currently believe is that adult implantees do need to learn how to interpret the new auditory cues being presented by the implant. ... If, for example, individuals spend little time in conversation, avoid contact with people, shop at the

supermarket, nod and smile in spite of not understanding, or talk all the time so that others can't get a word in edgewise, then they are spending very little time on task during their everyday lives and formal speech perception training in a rehab program will represent a dramatic increase. If, however, the individuals spend a good part of the day in meaningful spoken language exchanges, asking for repetitions if unsure, listening as well as talking, and taking on the challenge of communication under adverse conditions, then the additional time on task that can be offered within the constraints of a rehab program is small compared with the training they are giving themselves." (Personal communication, November 22, 1996. Used with permission.)

5. Vint Cerf, as quoted in Paula Bonillas, Lorraine Short, "Interview," *Hearing Health*, March/April 1997, p. 39.
6. Ludwig van Beethoven, "Heiligenstadt Testament," in *The Quiet Ear: Deafness in Literature*, comp. Brian Grant (London: Andre Deutsch, 1987), p. 71.
7. See the Resources listing for information on the *Learning to Hear Again* videotapes.
8. Kay Basham, "Love, Laughter, and Music," *CONTACT*, Summer 1993, p. 10.
9. Patricia A. Leake, "Long-Term Effects of Electrical Stimulation," *Program and Abstracts, NIH Consensus Development Conference, Cochlear Implants in Adults and Children*, Bethesda, Maryland, 1995, pp. 85-91.
10. D.B. Webster, M. Webster, "Neonatal Sound Deprivation Affects Brain Stem Auditory Nuclei," *Archives of Otolaryngology* 103 (1977): 392-96.
11. M.K. Schwaber et al., "Neuroplasticity of the Adult Primate Auditory Cortex Following Cochlear Hearing Loss," *American Journal of Otology* 14 (1993): 252-58.
12. Jean Moore and colleagues studied, postmortem, the temporal bones belonging to people who had become deaf as adults or teenagers. They confirmed that longer periods of deafness and

severe loss of peripheral ganglion cells had a more negative effect on the central auditory system than shorter periods of deafness and better survival of ganglion cells. However, Moore was surprised that there were many viable neurons present in the central auditory system for up to thirty years after onset of deafness. Jean K. Moore et al., "Effect of Adult-Onset Deafness on the Human Central Auditory System," *Annals of Otology, Rhinology & Laryngology* 106 (1997): 385-90.

13. Fan-Gang Zeng and Robert V. Shannon, researchers at the House Ear Institute in Los Angeles, postulate that the lower thresholds for low-frequency (bass) sounds observed in cochlear implant users might be due to the way in which low-frequency electrical impulses are actually processed by the brain. This processing might be different from the processing of high-frequency stimuli. Fan-Gang Zeng, Robert V. Shannon, "Loudness-Coding Mechanisms Inferred from Electric Stimulation of the Human Auditory System," *Science* 264 (1994): 564-66.

14. J.B. Nadol et al., "Survival of Spiral Ganglion Cells in Profound Sensorineural Hearing Loss: Implications for Cochlear Implantation," *Annals of Otology, Rhinology & Laryngology* 98 (1989): 411-16.

15. Peter Blamey, "Factors Affecting Auditory Performance of Postlingually Deaf Adults Using Cochlear Implants: Etiology, Age, and Duration of Deafness," *Program and Abstracts, NIH Consensus Development Conference, Cochlear Implants in Adults and Children*, Bethesda, Maryland, 1995, pp. 15-20. In spite of the findings that there are no correlations between spiral ganglion survival in the inner ear and performance with a cochlear implant, many scientists remain convinced there is a relationship. Some feel that the limiting factor in those cases studied postmortem may have actually been the device itself rather than neuronal survival. According to Robert Shannon, director of cochlear implant research at the House Ear Institute, researchers today simply do not fully understand the roles of

the inner ear spiral ganglions and the central auditory system in cochlear implant performance.

16. For a discussion of rates of improvements in deaf children with cochlear implants, see Dianne J. Allum-Mecklenburg, Gregorio Babighian, "Cochlear Implant Performance as an Indicator of Auditory Plasticity in Humans," in *Auditory System Plasticity and Regeneration*, ed. R.J. Salvi et al. (New York: Thieme, 1996).

17. Susan B. Waltzman et al., "Long-Term Results of Early Cochlear Implantation in Congenitally and Prelingually Deafened Children," *American Journal of Otology* 15 Suppl. 2 (1994): 9-13.

18. John K. Niparko et al., "Meta-Analysis of the Pediatric Cochlear Implant Literature," a paper delivered at the Fifth International Cochlear Implant Conference, New York, 1997 observed that "differences in performance diminish in time between congenital and acquired etiologies, and there is a distinct absence of plateauing of benefit over time."

19. Dianne J. Allum-Mecklenburg, Gregorio Babighian, "Cochlear Implant Performance as an Indicator of Auditory Plasticity in Humans," in *Auditory System Plasticity and Regeneration*, ed. R.J. Salvi et al. (New York: Thieme, 1996).

20. Patricia A. Leake, "Long-Term Effects of Electrical Stimulation," *Program and Abstracts, NIH Consensus Development Conference, Cochlear Implants in Adults and Children*, Bethesda, Maryland, 1995, pp. 85-91. See also: J. M. Miller et al., "Consequences of Deafness and Electrical Stimulation on the Auditory System," in *Auditory System Plasticity and Regeneration*, ed. R.J. Salvi et al. (New York: Thieme, 1996).

21. Leake and her colleagues determined that the cell size of a certain area of the cochlear nucleus of the brain that normally decreased drastically as a result of deafness showed less severe degeneration after a period of electrical stimulation.

22. J. Ito et al., "Positron Emission Tomography of Auditory Sensation in Deaf Patients and Patients with Cochlear Implants," *Annals of Otology, Rhinology & Laryngology* 102 (1993): 797-801.

23. Jane Shaw, "Switch On!" *CONTACT*, Summer 1992, p. 22.

24. Oliver Sacks, "To See and Not See," *New Yorker*, May 10, 1993. Also reprinted in *An Anthropologist on Mars* (Toronto: Alfred A. Knopf Canada, 1995).

25. G.H. Recanzone et al., "Plasticity in the Frequency Representation of Primary Auditory Cortex Following Discrimination Training in Adult Owl Monkeys," *Journal of Neuroscience* 13 (1993): 87-103.

26. Oliver Sacks, "To See and Not See," *New Yorker*, May 10, 1993, p. 70. Also reprinted in *An Anthropologist on Mars* (Toronto: Alfred A. Knopf Canada, 1995).

27. "Breakthroughs," *Discover*, July 1996. There is also some evidence that the auditory cortex may become devoted to other (possibly visual) tasks if it is not used for the learning of spoken language at the appropriate time, as pointed out by Susan Curtiss in "Issues in Language Acquisition Relevant to Cochlear Implants in Young Children," in *Cochlear Implants in Young Deaf Children*, ed. E. Owens and D.K. Kessler (Boston: College-Hill Press, 1989), p. 299.

28. G.H. Recanzone et al., "Topographic Reorganization of the Hand Representation in Cortical Area 3b Owl Monkeys Trained in a Frequency-Discrimination Task," *Journal of Neurophysiology*, 67 (1992): 1031-56.

29. A similar finding was made by R. Held as described by R.L. Gregory in *Eye and Brain* (New York: McGraw-Hill, 1966), p. 209. Held conducted an experiment on two kittens brought up in darkness. The only visual experience the kittens had was when they were placed in baskets as part of an experiment. The baskets were balanced on a beam so that one kitten was carried passively, and the other could move its own and the other kitten's basket through the movement of its limbs. The active kitten developed perceptual ability, but the passive one remained blind.

30. David Wright, *Deafness* (New York: Stein and Day, 1975), p. 12.

31. Oliver Sacks, "To See and Not See," *New Yorker*, May 10, 1993, p. 69. Also reprinted in *An Anthropologist on Mars* (Toronto: Alfred A. Knopf Canada, 1995).

32. See Dianne J. Allum, ed., *Cochlear Implant Rehabilitation in Children and Adults* (San Diego: Singular, 1996). In chapter after chapter, clinics from around the world report that some formal rehabilitation therapy is useful.

33. Ruth Oosterhof, in Beverly Biderman et al., "Roundtable Discussion: Learning to Listen with the CI," *CONTACT,* Summer 1996, p. 44.

34. Patricia A. Clickener, "How Can I Keep From Singing?" *SHHH Journal,* July/August 1993.

35. The 60% score is on the "HINT" (Hearing in Noise Test) that has become part of a standard battery of tests for adults, called the "Minimum Speech Test Battery." On the CID (Central Institute for the Deaf) sentence test, I score over 90%; on the CUNY (City University of New York) test I score around 70%. It is quite possible to become experienced on these sentence tests and to use skills other than hearing to figure them out. My monosyllabic word scores, however, remain the same regardless of the test, at around 30%. Audiologist Dorcas Kessler feels that the monosyllabic word tests are more reliable measures of hearing ability with cochlear implants and should be used instead of sentence tests.

36. For example, in a paper, "Speech Perception in Pediatric Cochlear Implant Recipients Receiving Total Communication, Oral and Auditory Verbal Training" presented at the Fifth International Cochlear Implant Conference, New York, 1997, S.D. Ash reported that "speech perception ability most closely correlates with the type of habilitative training received."

37. The Cochlear Implant Center in Hannover, Germany (Medinische Hochschule), for example, gives all parents of children with implants some training and guidance in auditory (re)habilitation.

38. Rather than sign and oral language being either/or propositions, they can co-exist, although a child with a cochlear implant still needs to be exposed to plenty of aural stimulation. Kessler and Owens state, "Numerous studies have demonstrated that the

acquisition and use of sign language in no way impedes, and may enhance, the development of other language skills, including speech production, lipreading, reading, and writing." ("Conclusions: Current Considerations and Future Directions," in *Cochlear Implants in Young Deaf Children*, ed. E. Owens and D.K. Kessler [Boston: College-Hill Press, 1989], p. 319.) See also Susan Curtiss, "Issues in Language Acquisition Relevant to Cochlear Implants in Young Children," in the same book. Curtiss points out that "there is an advantage to knowing *any* language over knowing no language during the preschool years" for the fostering of future spoken language and academic skills (p. 295). Curtiss also points out that deaf children of deaf parents, children who have learned ASL as their native language, can outperform deaf children of hearing parents on reading and writing tests, as well as on speech production measures (p. 295). In Sweden, training in sign language is a necessary criterion before a child receives a cochlear implant, and children are encouraged to maintain and develop their sign language skills after they get one. See: B. Aupeix et al., "Preoperative Selection According to a Psycho-Social Approach," a paper presented at the Fifth International Cochlear Implant Conference, New York, 1997. Also: "Differences between Adult and Child Rehabilitation Approaches: Auditory/Oral versus Signing/Speaking," in *Cochlear Implant Rehabilitation in Children and Adults*, ed. Dianne J. Allum (San Diego: Singular, 1996). The sign vs. oral controversy is a huge one that can only be touched upon briefly in this book.

39. Beverly Biderman, "Making Listening a Part of Children's Lives: An Interview with Warren Estabrooks," *CONTACT*, Fall 1995, p. 8.

40. Jane Meador, "Travels with Paige,"*CONTACT*, Summer 1991, p. 35.

41. In May of 1997, their mother sent me an update of the girls' test scores. Jessica, eleven months post-implant, at the age of 2.3 years scored at 2.0 years receptively and 1.6 years expressively. Rachel, seven years post-implant, at the age of nine years, and six months into grade 3 (grade 3.6), scored at the grade 3.8 level in reading comprehension, 3.1 level in vocabulary, and

5.6 level in language tests that included grammar, spelling, punctuation, and usage. Her overall grade level equivalency was 4.0. Jessica's test was administered by a certified auditory-verbal therapist, and Rachel's was the annual standardized test (Iowa Test of Basic Skills), administered to all the children in her (mainstream) class.

CHAPTER 3

1. Lou Ann Walker, *A Loss for Words: The Story of Deafness in a Family* (New York: Harper, 1986), p. 2. Walker is the hearing daughter of Deaf parents.

2. Bill Boyle, "The Implanted Iceman," *CONTACT*, Spring 1991, p. 5.

3. The damage potentially caused by hearing aids is still a concern to audiologists, because prolonged exposure to very loud sound, even in a damaged ear like mine, can cause permanent hearing loss. For example, in 1991, J.H. Macrae pointed out that for severe to profound losses, hearing aids that will be effective may also cause some permanent damage (J.H. Macrae, "Prediction of Deterioration in Hearing Due to Hearing Aid Use," *Journal of Speech and Hearing Research* 34 [1991]: 661-70). According to audiologist Dr. Charles Berlin, however, this damage may be preventable today with some of the relatively new fully digital programmable aids that have a wide dynamic range and follow the patient's loudness growth. He says these aids can strengthen the faint sounds that are inaudible to the patient, without boosting any of the loud sounds to a level that would cause damage. (Personal communication, June 1997.)

4. The end of World War II saw the return home of a large number of army veterans who became deaf from military noise exposure. The term "audiology" was coined in 1945, just a year before I was born. The first hearing aids that used transistors to partly replace cumbersome vacuum tubes did not appear until 1952, when I was six.

5. Note too, that no hearing aid can minutely analyze the frequency of incoming sounds and fine tune its response to them in the way a normal ear does.

6. Bonnie Poitras Tucker, *The Feel of Silence* (Philadelphia: Temple University Press, 1995), pp. 168-69.

7. "Decibel" is the term given to a relative measures of loudness, with 0 dB the arbitrarily defined reference point for the softest sound that the average normal ear can just barely detect about half the time.

8. Unidentified parent, as quoted in Roger Littleboy, "News from Australia," *TUNE-INternational*, Summer 1993.

9. Informal estimates from Gallaudet put the signing Deaf population in the United States at less than 500,000 out of an estimated total deaf population of 2 million. According to an informal estimate from the Canadian Hearing Society, the number of signing Deaf in Canada is approximately one-third of the total deaf population.

10. My average threshold was about 70 dB at the age of ten, and 115 dB by the time I got my implant.

11. The Canadian Hearing Society, *Hearing Loss: Questions and Answers*, May 1991, p. 2.

12. M. Leske, "Prevalence estimates of communicative disorders in the U.S.," *ASHA* 23 (1981): 229-327 as cited in J.G. Kyle et al., "Adjustment to Acquired Hearing Loss: A Working Model," in *Adjustment to Adult Hearing Loss*, ed. H. Orlans (San Diego: College-Hill Press, 1985), p. 119.

13. The Canadian Hearing Society, *Hearing Loss: Questions and Answers*, May 1991, p. 2; Canadian Hearing Society Bulletin CHS94102-05.

14. The Listening Center at Johns Hopkins, *Bringing Sound to Life for Deaf Children* (brochure).

15. The figure of 2 million profoundly deaf is cited in "Statistics on Deafness and Hearing Disorders in the United States," compiled and researched by the National Institute on Deafness and Other Communication Disorders (NIDCD), as reported in the *National Strategic Research Plan*, April 1988. The figure of 421,000 deaf in both ears is cited in the current (1997) "NIDCD Fact Sheet: Statistics on Deafness and Hearing

Disorders in the United States." For a breakdown of the number of deaf persons in the United States, which shows about 1 million who are deaf if the definition is "at best can hear and understand words shouted in the better ear," see *Demographic Aspects of Hearing Impairment: Questions and Answers* (Washington, D.C.: Gallaudet Research Institute, 1994).

16. Canadian Hearing Society (Bulletin CHS94102-05).

17. B.J.B. Keats et al., "Genetics and Hair Cell Loss," in *Hair Cells and Hearing Aids*, ed. C.I. Berlin (San Diego: Singular Publishing, 1996), p. 87: "The etiology of profound sensorineural hearing impairment in children is genetic in the majority of cases. Even when an environmental cause is indicated, predisposing genes are likely to play a significant role." Agnete Parving, however, in "Epidemiology of Genetic Hearing Impairment" in *Genetics and Hearing Impairment*, ed. A. Martini et al. (London: Whurr, 1996), writes that the proportion of genetic causes of hearing impairment (of all degrees) in childhood varies from 9 to 54% depending on the country. Professor Bronya Keats, the acting director of the Center for Molecular and Human Genetics at Louisiana State University Medical Center, says: "The confusion, and variability of estimates of the percentage of hearing impairment that is genetic, may arise from the fact that a genetic etiology does not imply a family history. In many families with only one hearing impaired child the cause is genetic, and genetic factors are likely to explain a large number of the cases for which the cause is classified as 'unknown'." (Personal communication, September 12, 1997. Used with permission.)

18. Oliver Sacks, *The Island of the Colorblind* (New York: Alfred A. Knopf, 1997), p. 239.

19. Adults and children who get cochlear implants may have become deaf due to a number of causes other than apparent hereditary factors. Some of these are meningitis, ototoxicity (an adverse reaction to drugs), otosclerosis, Meniere's dis-

ease, and viral infections. In many cases, the cause of deafness is unknown.

20. Kristin A. Buehl, from a message posted on the Internet CI Forum, November 11, 1997. Used with permission.

21. Lew Golan, *Reading Between the Lips: A Totally Deaf Man Makes It in the Mainstream* (Chicago: Bonus Books, 1995), p. 173.

22. P. Arnold, A. Kopsel, "Lipreading, Reading and Memory of Hearing and Hearing-Impaired Children," *Scandinavian Audiology* 25 (1996): 13-20.

23. R. Highfield, *Scientists Pay Lip Service to Language,* UK News Electronic Telegraph, 25 April, 1997. Reports on findings by British scientists using a brain scanner, that lipreading activates the auditory cortex. The possible implications of this are that good lipreaders might indeed do better with cochlear implants, and that good lipreaders can develop their skill from childhood.

24. S. B. Waltzman et al., "Predictors of Postoperative Performance with Cochlear Implants," in *Multicenter Comparative Study of Cochlear Implants: Final Reports of the Department of Veterans Affairs Cooperative Studies Program,* ed. N.L. Cohen and S.B. Waltzman, *Annals of Otology, Rhinology & Laryngology* 104 Suppl. 165 (1995): 15-18.

25. A. L. Perry and S. R. Silverman, "Speechreading," in *Hearing and Deafness,* ed. H. Davis and S.R. Silverman, Fourth Edition (New York: Holt, Rinehart and Winston, 1978), p. 385.

26. Ibid., p. 375.

27. One study using an automatic visual lipreading system was able to demonstrate a 47% accuracy in understanding speech (not just phonemes) based only on video images and automated rules. P.L. Silsbee, A.C. Bovik, "Automatic Lipreading," *Biomedical Sciences Instrumentation* 29 (1993): 415-22.

28. H. Davis, "Audiometry: Pure-Tone and Simple Speech Tests," in *Hearing and Deafness,* ed. H. Davis and S.R. Silverman, Fourth Edition (New York: Holt, Rinehart and Winston, 1978), p. 217.

29. In France, some children use Cued Speech before getting an

implant to improve their language proficiency, and then in the early period of using the device, learn to make the proper connections between what is seen and what is heard, and eventually drop the cueing.

30. Harry G. Lang, *Silence of the Spheres: the Deaf Experience in the History of Science* (Westport, Connecticut: Bergin & Garvey, 1994), pp. 70-71.

31. Ibid., p. 63.

32. J.M. Weisenberger, M.E. Percy, "Use of the Tactaid II and Tactaid VII With Children," in *The Effectiveness of Cochlear Implants and Tactile Aids for Deaf Children: The Sensory Aids Study at Central Institute for the Deaf*, ed. A.E. Geers and J.S. Moog, *Volta Review* 96 (1994): 41-57.

33. Evelyn Glennie, as quoted in Andrew Solomon, "Defiantly Deaf," *New York Times Magazine*, August 28, 1994, p. 44.

34. Evelyn Glennie, *Good Vibrations* (Long Preston, North Yorkshire, England: Magna Print Books, 1990), p. 180.

35. D.A. Ramsdell, "The Psychology of the Hard-of-Hearing and the Deafened Adult," in *Hearing and Deafness*, ed. H. Davis and S.R. Silverman, Fourth Edition (New York: Holt, Rinehart and Winston, 1978).

36. Ramsdell says that this overwhelming feeling of being not just deaf, but dead can afflict those adults who become deafened suddenly and those who like me become deaf gradually. It is unlikely to affect those who are born profoundly deaf and never had this auditory link with their surroundings (ibid., p. 507).

37. Joanne Syrja, "My Cochlear Implant Made Me FAT!" *CONTACT*, Spring 1993, p. 21.

38. K.P. Meadow-Orlans, "Social and Psychological Effects of Hearing Loss in Adulthood: A Literature Review," in *Adjustment to Adult Hearing Loss*, ed. H. Orlans (San Diego: College-Hill Press, 1985), p. 40.

39. Anthony Storr, *Music and the Mind* (New York: The Free Press, 1992), p. 26.

40. Celeste Coleon, personal communication, January 15, 1997. Used with permission.

41. M. Vernon et al., "Hearing Loss," *SHHH Journal,* March/April 1982.

42. C.P. Shah et al., "Delay in Referral of Children with Impaired Hearing," *Volta Review* 80 (1978): 207 as cited in the *Ontario Medical Review,* May 1993, p. 46.

43. The U.S. National Institutes of Health 1993 Consensus Development Conference on Early Identification of Hearing Impairment in Infants and Young Children warned that parental concern about a child's hearing should be sufficient reason to initiate prompt formal hearing evaluation.

CHAPTER 4

1. David Wright, *Deafness* (New York: Stein and Day, 1975), p. 5.

2. David M. Luterman with Mark Ross, *When Your Child Is Deaf* (Parkton: York Press, 1991), p. 3.

3. Statistics on oral deaf-hearing marriages are difficult to find. Jerome Schein found that in Metropolitan Washington, D.C., the percentage of divorces among hearing-and-deaf couples was disproportionately high. His population of deaf people, however, included both oral deaf and signing Deaf persons. Jerome D. Schein, *The Deaf Community: Studies in the Social Psychology of Deafness* (Washington, D.C.: Gallaudet College Press, 1968).

4. Frank Martin, "The Impact of a Cochlear Implant on a Partner," *CONTACT,* Summer 1995, p. 6.

5. Pauline Ashley, "Deafness and the Family," in *Adjustment to Adult Hearing Loss,* ed. H. Orlans (San Diego: College-Hill Press, 1985).

6. David Wright, *Deafness* (New York: Stein and Day, 1975), p. 111.

7. Jos Patel, "A Spouse's Story," *CONTACT,* Spring 1994, p. 7.

8. Pauline Ashley, "Deafness and the Family," in *Adjustment to Adult Hearing Loss,* ed. H. Orlans (San Diego: College-Hill Press, 1985).

9. Donna L. Sorkin, "An Odyssey Through Hearing Loss: A Personal Perspective on Cochlear Implants," *SHHH Journal*, January/February 1994, p. 17.

10. J.A. Beattie "Social Aspects of Acquired Hearing Loss in Adults," unpublished Ph.D. thesis, 1981, University of Bradford, as cited in *Words Apart: Losing Your Hearing as an Adult*, Leslie Jones et al. (London: Tavistock, 1987), p. 191.

11. Harold Orlans and Kathryn P. Meadow-Orlans, "Responses to Hearing Loss: Effects on Social Life, Leisure, and Work," *SHHH Journal*, January/February 1985.

12. Ruth Sidransky, *In Silence: Growing up Hearing in a Deaf World* (New York: Ballantine, 1990), p. 153.

13. Eve Nickerson, "Taking Control and Letting Go," in Kay Thomsett and Eve Nickerson, *Missing Words: The Family Handbook on Adult Hearing Loss* (Washington, D.C.: Gallaudet University Press, 1993), p. 98.

14. Bob Biderman, "A Workshop for Spouses of Cochlear Implant Users," *CONTACT*, Summer/Fall 1997.

15. Kathy Urschel, "The Impulse to Soar," *CONTACT*, Summer 1996, p. 9.

CHAPTER 5

1. Samuel Johnson, *A Journey to the Western Islands of Scotland*, excerpted in *The Quiet Ear: Deafness in Literature*, comp. B. Grant (London: Andre Deutsch, 1987), p. 15. Johnson was writing about his visit to a school for deaf children in Edinburgh, Scotland.

2. Paula Bartone-Bonillas, "Out of Sound," *Hearing Health*, June/July 1992, p. 19.

3. Caitlin Parton, in Paula Bonillas, "Listen to the Children," *Hearing Health*, August/September 1993, p. 29.

4. Methods have been developed, however, to implant ossified (bone-filled) cochleae. Dr. Thomas Balkany, speaking at the Fifth International Cochlear Implant Conference, 1997, New York, declared that "total ossification is no longer a contraindi-

cation" for cochlear implant surgery ("Further Developments in Implantation of the Obstructed Cochlea").

5. Five years later, in 1997, the average score at the clinic for the same test with a much larger group was around 80%.

6. See for example, R. S. Tyler, N. Tye-Murray, "Cochlear Implant Signal-Processing Strategies and Patient Perception of Speech and Environmental Sounds," in *Cochlear Implants: A Practical Guide,* ed. Huw Cooper (San Diego: Singular, 1991), p. 73.

7. Mardie Younglof, from a message posted on the Internet CI Forum, July 18, 1997. Used with permission.

8. Oliver Sacks, "To See and Not See," *New Yorker,* May 10, 1993. Also reprinted in *An Anthropologist on Mars* (Toronto: Alfred A. Knopf Canada, 1995).

9. For example, J.G. Toner of Ireland has performed cochlear implant surgery under local anaesthetic. J. G. Toner, R. Stewart, "Implant Surgery under Local Anaesthesia: Implications for Patient Selection," presentation at the Fifth International Cochlear Implant Conference, New York, 1997.

10. In 1988, the first detailed report of surgical complications of cochlear implant surgery indicated 55 complications out of 459 implant operations, yielding an overall incidence of 11.8%. The most common problem was infection of the cut skin flap behind the ear. N.L. Cohen et al., "Medical or Surgical Complications Related to the Nucleus Multichannel Cochlear Implant," *Annals of Otology, Rhinology, & Laryngology* 97 Suppl. 135 (1988): 8-13. In 1995, a report showed an overall rate of 12.2% if device failure was included, and 9.8% if device failure was excluded (i.e., leaving only surgical complications). R. A. Hoffman, N. L. Cohen, "Complications of Cochlear Implant Surgery," *Proceedings of the International Cochlear Implant, Speech and Hearing Symposium* (Melbourne, 1994), p. 420. A study of 309 children showed 12 (3.9%) had major complications that required either surgery or intravenous antibiotics, and a study of 548 children showed 9 (2.9%) had minor complications of surgery: G. M. Clark et al., "Surgical and Safety Considerations

of Multi-channel Cochlear Implants in Children," *Ear and Hearing*, Vol. 12, No. 4, Suppl. (1991): 15S-24S as cited in *Cochlear Implantation for Infants and Children: Advances*, ed. G. M. Clark et al. (San Diego: Singular Publishing, 1997), p. 122.

11. W. M. Luxford, D. E. Brackmann, "The History of Cochlear Implants," in *Cochlear Implants*, ed. R.F. Gray (London: Croom Helm, 1985), p. 1.

12. Ibid., p. 2.

13. F. Blair Simmons, "History of Cochlear Implants in the United States: A Personal Perspective," in *Cochlear Implants*, ed. R.A. Schindler, M.M. Merzenich (New York: Raven Press, 1985), p. 4.

14. J.M. Syrja, "Anatomy of an Implant," *CONTACT*, Fall 1993, p. 6.

15. Jim Patrick, personal communication, May 2, 1997.

16. Graeme Clark, personal communication, May 15, 1997. Used with permission.

17. Attempts have been made to develop a visual prosthesis for the blind based on electrodes similar to those of a cochlear implant; however, an effective device to give blind people usable vision may still be far off. See for example, E. M. Schmidt et al., "Feasibility of a Visual Prosthesis for the Blind Based on Intracortical Microstimulation of the Visual Cortex," *Brain* 119 (1996): 507-522. The study reported that a blind patient was able to see small spots of light as a result of stimulation of temporary electrodes implanted in her visual cortex, but little more than that.

18. Dorcas K. Kessler, "Cochlear Implants: Past, Present, and Future," *CONTACT*, Winter 1992, p. 10.

19. J. Muller et al., "Evaluation of Performance with the Combi 40 in Adults: A Multicenter Clinical Study," paper presented at the Fifth International Cochlear Implant Conference, New York, 1997.

20. R.C. Dowell et al., "Potential and Limitations of Cochlear Implants in Children," *Proceedings of the International Cochlear Implant, Speech and Hearing Symposium* (Melbourne, 1994).

21. Richard C. Dowell, Robert S.C. Cowan, "Evaluation of Benefit: Infants and Children," in *Cochlear Implantation for Infants and*

Children: Advances, ed. G. M. Clark et al. (San Diego: Singular Publishing, 1997).

22. T. Serry et al., " Phoneme Acquisition in the First Four Years of Implant Use," paper presented at the Third European Symposium on Paediatric Cochlear Implantation, Hannover, Germany, 1996. Cited in Richard C. Dowell, Robert S.C. Cowan, "Evaluation of Benefit: Infants and Children," in *Cochlear Implantation for Infants and Children: Advances,* ed. G. M. Clark et al. (San Diego: Singular Publishing, 1997).

23. Shirley and Julian Keller, "Dara," in *Auditory-Verbal Therapy for Parents and Professionals,* ed. Warren Estabrooks (Washington, D.C.: Alexander Graham Bell Association for the Deaf, 1994), p. 177.

24. Nottingham Paediatric Cochlear Implant Programme, *Progress Report: Outcomes for Paediatric Cochlear Implantation in Nottingham: Safe, Effective, Efficient,* May 1997. For a copy of the report, contact the Nottingham Paediatric Cochlear Implant Programme, 113 The Ropewalk, Nottingham NG1 6HA, England.

25. M.J. Osberger, "Clinical Investigation of the CLARION Multi-Strategy Cochlear Implant in Children," paper presented at the Fifth International Cochlear Implant Conference, New York, 1997. See also the more detailed analysis of the first thirty-nine children in the group (the analysis showed significant improvements over time on all test scores): M.J. Osberger et al., "Clinical Results with the CLARION Multi-strategy Cochlear Implant in Children," in *Cochlear Implants: XVI World Congress of Otorhinolaryngology Head and Neck Surgery, Sydney (Australia), 1997: Cochlear Implants,* ed. G.M. Clark (Bologna: Monduzzi Editore, 1996).

26. Graeme Clark, "Media Release November 25, 1996: New Generation of Electrodes: A New Era in Bionic Ears," *CICADA Vic,* February 1997, p. 4.

27. But see A. Zhang et al., "The Development of a Tympanic Membrane Sensor for a Totally Implantable Cochlear Implant

or Hearing Aid," in *Cochlear Implants: XVI World Congress of Otorhinolaryngology Head and Neck Surgery, Sydney (Australia), 1997: Cochlear Implants*, ed. G.M. Clark (Bologna: Monduzzi Editore, 1996).

28. The first time a deaf person received a single-channel ABI was in 1979, at the House Ear Institute (HEI) in Los Angeles. The first time a deaf person received a multichannel ABI (which represented an advance over the single-channel one) was in 1992, also at the HEI.

29. John Petito, "When the Brain Hears," *CONTACT*, Spring 1992, p. 10.

30. Steven R. Otto et al., "Coinvestigator Results with the Multi-channel Auditory Brainstem Implant," paper presented at the Fifth International Cochlear Implant Conference, New York, 1997.

31. Dorcas K. Kessler, "Cochlear Implants: Past, Present, and Future," *CONTACT*, Winter 1992, pp. 11, 12.

32. In 1996, in the paper "Cochlear Implants: Patient Selection and Preoperative Assessment," presented at the Asia Pacific Symposium on Cochlear Implant, Kyoto, 1996, Pierre Montandon and Marco Pelizzone reported on the huge variability of scores even when individuals were provided with an upgrade (from compressed analog to continuous interleaved sampling) but using the same device (the Ineraid, which is no longer produced). They concluded that about 80% of the variance in scores across individuals was related not to the processing strategy, but to individual factors associated with the implant user. Moreover, it was not clear as to what those individual factors were, since auditory brainstem responses did not reveal much correspondence between likely nerve survival and performance.

33. Peter Seligman, "Lucky Coincidences," *CONTACT*, Spring 1993, p. 22.

34. Although candidates are warned to expect the destruction of residual hearing in the implanted ear, more than one study has found that residual hearing can be preserved, even in the case

of the deep electrode array insertion of multichannel implants. In this study, conservation of hearing occurred in 52% of a group of forty patients: A. Hodges et al., "Conservation of Residual Hearing with Cochlear Implantation," *American Journal of Otology* 18 (1997): 179-83. Dr. William House, a pioneer Californian surgeon in the cochlear implant field, and owner of a U.S. company manufacturing single-electrode devices, is a strong proponent of single-electrode implants, believing that the fact their insertion is less traumatic to the inner ear is a major point in their favor.

35. Nancy Hoffmann, personal communication, June 9, 1997. Used with permission.

36. Chris Arcia, "ABI Party Tricks," *CONTACT*, Summer 1994, p. 7 .

37. "Baptism of Fire." Copyright 1979 Julie Snow Music, BMI. Used with permission.

CHAPTER 6

1. Carol Padden and Tom Humphries, *Deaf in America* (Cambridge, Massachusetts: Harvard University Press, 1988), p. 44. The authors are themselves members of the Deaf culture.

2. For example, in American Sign Language, there are around 3,000 root signs, which when combined with the large number of possible movements of the signer's body for grammatical differentiation, allow for rich and complex expression. There are literally hundreds of variations of the root sign "look" including "stare," "gaze," "watch," " look for a long time," "look at incessantly," and so forth. William Stokoe, discussing the number of ASL signs, says, "A sign language sign is not the same thing as a word, it is only an artifact of someone's attempt to partition off parts of a visible flow. If handshape and movement only are considered and the facial and other non-manual activity ignored, the undercounting will be extreme. ... Every language is perfectly adequate to express whatever its users, the sharers of its culture, need and want to express with it." (Personal communication, August 22, 1997. Used with permission.)

3. William C. Stokoe, *Sign Language Structure* (Buffalo: Dept. of Anthropology and Linguistics, University of Buffalo, 1960).

4. The modern-day plight of deaf children in Berundi, who generally receive no education and are considered ineducable, is described in Harlan Lane et al., *A Journey into the DEAF-WORLD* (San Diego: DAWNSIGNPRESS, 1996), p. 192.

5. Oliver Sacks, *Seeing Voices* (Berkeley and Los Angeles: University of California Press, 1989), pp. 53-54.

6. Judith A. Holt, "Stanford Achievement Test – 8th Edition: Reading Comprehension Subgroup Results," *American Annals of the Deaf*, April, 1993. The subsequent ninth edition analysis, prepared in 1996, avoided averaging scores to obtain "overall" scores, stating that such an averaging ignored the fact that the students being averaged were taking different levels of the Stanford Tests as well as achieving different scores. Instead of a gross average, a ranking of deaf and hard-of-hearing students that used percentiles was presented. Using this ranking, deaf and hard-of-hearing students were compared with other deaf and hard-of-hearing students instead of hearing students. *Stanford Achievement Test, 9th Edition, Form S, Norms Booklet for Deaf and Hard-of-Hearing Students* (Washington, D.C.: Gallaudet Research Institute, 1996).

7. Kathryn Woodcock, "Yes, We Have No Implants," *CONTACT,* Spring 1993, p. 37.

8. *Le Pays des Sourds*, France, 1992, directed by Nicolas Philibert.

9. Contrast his wish for a deaf child with Alexander Graham Bell's view that the tendency of the deaf to marry other deaf people was an "evil" since it tended to produce a "deaf variety of the human race." Bell's prescription was to reduce the segregation of the deaf and to educate them with hearing children. Alexander Graham Bell, *Memoirs Upon the Formation of a Deaf Variety of the Human Race* (New Haven: National Academy of Science, 1883).

10. Gordon L. Nystedt, from a message posted on the Internet CI Forum, June 1, 1997. Used with permission.

11. Charlene LeBlanc, as quoted in Carol Milstone, "Sound and Fury," *Saturday Night*, March 1996, p. 25.

12. Canadian Association of the Deaf, Press Release, January 25, 1994.

13. "The Use of Cochlear Implants," *Silent News*, June 1991.

14. Judith Treesberg, as quoted in Carol Milstone, "Sound and Fury," *Saturday Night*, March 1996, p. 26.

15. J.R. Wyatt et al., "Cost Effectiveness of the Multichannel Cochlear Implant," *American Journal of Otology* 16 (1995): 52-62.

16. In Australia, the costs for educating deaf children in special schools have been placed at $25,039 each per year, in contrast to the cost of $4,420 per primary student and $6,461 per secondary student in regular schools. In the United States, savings of $152,000 in educational costs for each child implanted at the age of four have been cited. For a discussion, see Robert S.C. Cowan, "Socioeconomic and Educational Management Issues," in *Cochlear Implantation for Infants and Children: Advances*, ed. G.M. Clark et al. (San Diego: Singular Publishing, 1997).

17. Diane Marleau, Minister of National Health and Welfare, Canada, correspondence with the author, July 21, 1994.

18. "Cochlear Implants in Children: A Position Paper of the National Association of the Deaf," *The NAD Broadcaster*, March 1991, p. 1.

19. Larry Orloff, "Editor's Message," *CONTACT*, Winter 1996, p. 11.

20. *CAD CHAT*, June 1994.

21. Sarah Butler, from a message posted on the CompuServe online Disabilities Forum, Deaf/Hard of Hearing Section, February 18, 1997. Used with permission.

22. J.D. McCaughey, "Cochlear Implants: Some Considerations of a More or Less Ethical Character," *Proceedings of the International Cochlear Implant Speech and Hearing Symposium* (Melbourne, 1994), p. 16. For a comprehensive treatment of the ethics of cochlear implantation in children as related to the Helsinki Declaration on Biomedical Research, see G. M. Clark et al., "Ethical Issues," in *Cochlear Implantation for Infants and Children: Advances*, ed. G.M. Clark et al. (San Diego: Singular Publishing, 1997).

23. Beverly Biderman, "Building Bridges: An Interview with Gary Malkowski," *CONTACT*, Winter-Spring 1995.

24. Rick Apicella, personal communication, November 22, 1996. Used with permission.

25. R. E. West, J. Stucky, "Cochlear Implantation Outcomes: Experience with the Nucleus 22 Channel Implant," *Proceedings of the International Cochlear Implant Speech and Hearing Symposium* (Melbourne 1994), p. 447.

26. Darrell E. Rose, "Cochlear Implants in Children With Prelingual Deafness: Another Side of the Coin," *American Journal of Audiology* 3 (1994): 6. In the final report on the study, Rose and his colleagues obtained results from forty-five of sixty-four residential and day schools for the deaf, including three with oral programs. Of the 151 implanted children identified, only 53% of the children were wearing their units on a regular basis, but not surprisingly, 65% of these children were in the three schools with oral programs. Fifty out of the fifty-two children with implants in the oral programs were using their implants. The study's authors suggested that the candidate selection process for prelingually deaf children might be faulty, and children with implants needed access to strong aural/oral programs. D.E. Rose et al., "Cochlear Implants in Prelingually Deaf Children," *American Annals of the Deaf* 141 (1996): 258-261.

27. R. E. West, J. Stucky, "Cochlear Implantation Outcomes: Experience with the Nucleus 22 Channel Implant," *Proceedings of the International Cochlear Implant Speech and Hearing Symposium* (Melbourne 1994), p. 448.

28. Margery N. Somers, "Effects of Cochlear Implants in Children: Implications for Rehabilitation," in *Cochlear Implants: A Practical Guide*, ed. Huw Cooper (San Diego: Singular Publishing, 1991), p. 330. Somers cites 1987 and 1990 reports to support a finding that 9% of children with cochlear implants are mainstreamed. P.M. Chute, in 1997, reports a much higher rate. P.M. Chute et al., "Educational Achievements of Children with Cochlear Implants," a paper presented at the Fifth

International Cochlear Implant Conference, New York, 1997, reported that of ninety-two children with cochlear implants followed by the Manhattan Eye, Ear and Throat Hospital in New York, more than 50% of the children implanted between the ages of two and four were placed in mainstream educational settings within two years of implantation; by seven years post-implantation, all ninety-two children were being educated in the mainstream.

29. Brent Sunderland, as quoted in Marie Arana-Ward, "As Technology Advances, a Bitter Debate Divides the Deaf," *Washington Post*, May 11, 1997, Page A1.

30. Elaine Burak, "Adolescents Offer Challenge," *CONTACT*, Spring 1992, pp. 6-7. The problem of some teenagers giving up their cochlear implants, even when they seem to be benefitting from the device, is well documented. Carmen Pujol and Teresa Amat of Spain make a perceptive observation when they say, "The biggest challenge with adolescent cochlear implant patients is not whether they will utilize auditory sensations effectively, but whether they will identify themselves as hearing individuals." Carmen Pujol, Teresa Amat, "Adolescents and the Cochlear Implant," in *Cochlear Implant Rehabilitation in Children and Adults*, ed. Dianne J. Allum (San Diego: Singular Publishing, 1996).

31. John F. Knutson, "Psychological and Social Issues in Cochlear Implant Use," *Program and Abstracts, NIH Consensus Development Conference, Cochlear Implants in Adults and Children*, Bethesda, Maryland, 1995, p. 68.

32. Noel Cohen, a cochlear implant surgeon at New York University Medical Center, for example, states, "Much has been made of the comparison between cochlear implant surgery and tonsillectomy and adenoidectomy, but this is actually a very favorable comparison, since the risk of tonsillectomy and adenoidectomy is greatly underestimated, and on occasion leads to fatal complications. There has never been a cochlear implant-related death." In "Medical and Surgical Perspectives: Issues in Treatment and Management of Severe and Profound Hearing

Impairment," *Proceedings, International Cochlear Implant, Speech and Hearing Symposium* (Melbourne, 1994), p. 150.

33. Harlan Lane, "Cochlear Implants Are Wrong for Young Deaf Children," *The NAD Broadcaster,* March 1992.

34. Lane and his co-authors make the same point against cochlear implants in Harlan Lane et al., *A Journey into the DEAF-WORLD* (San Diego: DAWNSIGNPRESS, 1996).

35. Caitlin Parton, "60 Minutes," CBS Television News, November 8, 1992.

36. "60 Minutes," CBS Television News, November 8, 1992.

37. Michelle Smithdas, "Piercing My Silent World," *CONTACT,* Winter-Spring 1995, p. 15.

38. M.M. Cohen Jr., R.J. Gorlin, "Epidemiology, Etiology, and Genetic Patterns," in *Hereditary Hearing Loss and its Syndromes,* R.J. Gorlin et al. (New York: Oxford University Press, 1995). Jerome Schein postulates a "90-percent rule of deaf family life:" 90 percent of deaf children have hearing parents; 90 percent of deaf adults marry someone deaf; 90 percent of children born to deaf parents are hearing. Jerome D. Schein, *At Home Among Strangers* (Washington, D.C.: Gallaudet University Press, 1989), p. 106.

39. Dawn Walker, in Paula Bonillas, "Listen to the Children," *Hearing Health,* August/September 1993, p. 27.

40. Helmut L. Neumann, Renate Meixner, "A Psycholinguistic Approach to the Rehabilitation of Cochlear Implant Children," in *Cochlear Implant Rehabilitation in Children and Adults,* ed. Dianne J. Allum (San Diego: Singular Publishing, 1996).

41. Emily Perl Kingsley, "Kids Like These," from the teleplay produced for CBS Television by Nexus Publications Inc. and Taft Entertainment, as cited in David M. Luterman with Mark Ross, *When Your Child Is Deaf: A Guide for Parents* (Parkton, Maryland: York Press, 1991), p. 78.

42. Max Blum, "David," in *Auditory-Verbal Therapy for Parents and Professionals,* ed. Warren Estabrooks (Washington, D.C.: Alexander Graham Bell Association for the Deaf, 1994), p. 186.

43. Some Deaf culture advocates believe that hearing parents are not

getting enough information about the choice they have to leave their child's deafness alone, and allow the child to become part of the Deaf culture. While this may be true in some cases, many clinics do try to provide information about the Deaf culture option to parents. The cochlear implant team at Toronto's Hospital for Sick Children, for example, gives parents investigating a cochlear implant for their child a handbook that contains the statements of the Ontario Association of the Deaf (opposing the implant and offering information about Deaf culture) along with statements from other groups that point out the efficacy of the device.

CHAPTER 7

1. Heather Whitestone, Miss America 1995, is profoundly deaf and lost her hearing at the age of eighteen months as a result of the complications of whooping cough. She was widely proclaimed as the "first person with a disability" to hold the title of Miss America. Miss Whitestone is oral deaf, and a graduate of auditory-verbal therapy.

2. See for example, Glen Golightly, Lisa Teachery, "Misunderstanding Leads to Murder," in *Silent News*, April 1994, p. 12, for the story of a deaf and mute man in Houston, Texas, who was shot and killed when he apparently did not understand a robber's demand for his money. Also: Brenda Ingersoll, "Deaf Patron Scraps with Gunman," in *Silent News*, November 1996. The report starts out this way: "Rodney Schilleman is Deaf, so he didn't hear a gunman order everyone at Stevens restaurant to stay on the floor for five minutes in 'spread-eagle' position after a robbery Thursday." Schilleman of Madison, Wisconsin, survived a beating by the robber.

3. Angelica Carranza, "Follow Your Dream," *CONTACT*, Fall 1994, p. 20.

4. D.J. Allum-Mecklenburg, G. Babighian, "Cochlear Implant Performance as an Indicator of Auditory Plasticity in Humans," in *Auditory System Plasticity and Regeneration*, ed. R.J. Salvi et al. (New York: Thieme, 1996).

5. Patricia A. Leake, "Long-Term Effects of Electrical Stimulation," *Program and Abstracts, NIH Consensus Development Conference, Cochlear Implants in Adults and Children*, Bethesda, Maryland, 1995, pp. 85-91. See also: J. M. Miller et al., "Consequences of Deafness and Electrical Stimulation on the Auditory System," in *Auditory System Plasticity and Regeneration*, ed. R.J. Salvi et al. (New York: Thieme, 1996).

6. A good lay discussion of ear hair cell regeneration is found in the open-captioned video and accompanying printed transcript for "Hair Cell Regeneration: We've Come a Long Way in a Few Short Years" by Edwin Rubel (Self Help for Hard of Hearing People Inc. [SHHH], 1994). May be ordered from SHHH at 7910 Woodmont Avenue, Suite 1200, Bethesda, MD 20814. More technical discussions are found in *Auditory System Plasticity and Regeneration*, ed. R.J. Salvi et al. (New York: Thieme, 1996).

7. Edwin Rubel, "Hair Cell Regeneration: We've Come a Long Way in a Few Short Years."

8. Edwin Rubel, personal communication, June 24, 1997. Used with permission.

9. Brenda Morgan Ryals, personal communication, July 22, 1997. Used with permission.

10. See J. D. Green Jr. et al., "Binaural Cochlear Implants," *American Journal of Otology* 13 (1992): 502-06. In a study of just six binaural cochlear implant users, performance for some was better in binaural conditions, but according to the study's authors, the improvements were not great.

11. Dianne J. Allum-Mecklenburg, personal communication, June 28, 1997.

12. Some cochlear implant clinics, including the House Ear Clinic in Los Angeles, recommend that patients keep wearing a hearing aid in the non-implanted ear if possible.

13. B.S. Kou et al., "Subjective Benefits Reported by Adult Nucleus 22-Channel Cochlear Implant Users," *Journal of Otolaryngology* 23 (1994): 8-14.

14. A. Hogan, "Measures of Psycho-Social Outcomes in Adult Cochlear Implant Programs," in *Sixteenth World Congress of Otorhinolaryngology Head and Neck Surgery, Sydney (Australia), 1997: Cochlear Implants,* ed. G.M. Clark (Bologna: Monduzzi Editore, 1996).

15. Celeste Coleon, personal communication, January 15, 1997. Used with permission.

16. G. M. Clark, untitled foreword, in *Cochlear Implants: Sixteenth World Congress of Otorhinolaryngology Head and Neck Surgery, Sydney (Australia), 1997: Cochlear Implants,* ed. G.M. Clark (Bologna: Monduzzi Editore, 1996).

17. S.S. Graham, J.R.E. Dickins, "Current Demographic Characteristics of Cochlear Implant Children in the United States," *Annals of Otology, Rhinology and Laryngology* 104 Suppl. 166 (1995): 240-43. The report states that of 17,634 profoundly deaf children identified in the United States, 1,844 had cochlear implants as of July 1, 1994. There were 513 children in the United States between the ages of two and five who had implants, representing 21% of the profoundly deaf children identified in this age group. These figures indicate a significant potential impact on the education of deaf children in the United States.

18. Ron West, president and CEO, Cochlear Corporation, personal communication, June 12, 1997.

19. Douglas P. Lynch, manager of public relations, Advanced Bionics Corporation, personal communication, July 31, 1997.

20. *Prospectus,* Cochlear Limited, October 24, 1995.

21. Joanne Syrja, the manager of reimbursement services for Advanced Bionics Corporation, says, "Health care is a competitive arena. Cochlear implants are a low volume surgical procedure. As such, many payers do not give cochlear implants the reimbursement status of a prosthesis and the automatic pre-authorization for payment they deserve. Medical reviewers at the insurers still need to be educated about cochlear implants." (Personal communication, August 27, 1997. Used with permission.) See also: Joanne Syrja, "Cochlear Implants: Who Pays

and How Much?" a presentation at the Fifth International Cochlear Implant Conference, New York, 1997.

22. Sue Archbold, "Implant Centre and Teachers of the Deaf: Conflict or Collaboration?" a paper presented at the Fifth International Cochlear Implant Conference, New York, 1997.

23. G.J. Dooley et al., "Combined Electrical and Acoustical Stimulation Using a Bimodal Prosthesis," *Archives of Otolaryngology – Head & Neck Surgery* 119 (1993): 55-60. Also: J.K. Shallop, "Research Note: The Bimodal Speech Processor," *CONTACT*, Summer 1993, p. 25.

24. Nancy Hoffmann, "Living with Koalas and Baby Butcherbirds," *CONTACT*, Winter 1996, p. 32.

25. Noel Cohen, interview, New York, May 1, 1997.

26. See the survey: Fan-Gang Zeng, "Cochlear Implants in Developing Countries," *CONTACT*, Winter 1996, p. 5. This survey includes a discussion of the low-cost implant system under development at the House Ear Institute.

27. At the Fifth International Cochlear Implant Conference in New York City, 1997, the issue of the cost of cochlear implant equipment came up. When asked for his "wish list" to present to device manufacturers, Dr. Noel Cohen asked why cochlear implants couldn't be like computers. Computers, he said, are increasing in complexity, while their costs are declining. Cochlear implants, on the other hand, are getting both more complex, and more expensive. When I later contacted Cochlear Corporation president and CEO, Ron West, for a response to this, he pointed out that the volume of sales of cochlear implants simply does not allow for the economy of scale permitted to computer manufacturers. Moreover, expenses are high: he estimated that a company developing a new cochlear implant system today in the United States can expect to invest the staggering sum of $30 to $40 million to cover the rigorous testing and FDA approval process required before commercial sale of the device.

28. Gary E. Mowl, "Raising Deaf Children in Hearing Society:

Struggles and Challenges for Deaf Native ASL Signers," in *Cultural and Language Diversity and the Deaf Experience,* ed. Ila Parasnis (Cambridge: Cambridge University Press, 1996), pp. 233-34.

29. Larry Orloff, "Editor's Message," *CONTACT,* Fall 1993, p. 33.

30. K. Fishman et al., "Speech Recognition as a Function of the Number of Electrodes Used in the Speak Cochlear Implant Speech Processor," *Journal of Speech and Hearing Research,* in press, 1997. The performance of the subjects improved as the number of electrodes activated was increased from one to seven, but then, strangely, there was no change as the number of active electrodes was increased from seven to twenty. Although these findings are interesting, care should be taken in interpreting them. The subjects in the study all had at least nineteen active electrodes available for activation. Dr. Noel Cohen, for example, notes that clinically, patients with as few as six electrodes activated, in systems with twenty-two electrodes, will typically not do as well as the group will do as a whole (personal communication, September 2, 1997). Having more electrodes may present an advantage, moreover, in that it can give the clinician a larger set of electrodes from which to select the appropriate ones to activate. Picking these, however, is not always easy.

31. R.V. Shannon, "Cochlear Implants: What Have We Learned and Where Are We Going?" *Seminars in Hearing* 17 (1996): 403-15.

EPILOGUE

1. David M. Luterman with Mark Ross, *When Your Child Is Deaf: A Guide for Parents* (Parkton, Maryland: York Press, 1991), p. 13.

2. "Baptism of Fire." Copyright 1979 Julie Snow Music, BMI. Used with permission.

RESOURCES

What follows is a non-exhaustive list of resources that may be useful to those who wish more information about cochlear implants, or about deafness and hearing impairments in general. It is but a sampling of a larger set of resources too numerous to list – for example, there are many centers for research into cochlear implants at universities around the world.

Please note also that the information is subject to change, especially in the case of electronic mail and World Wide Web (WWW) addresses. You may need to call or write to confirm an electronic address, and responses via e-mail may not always be prompt.

Phone and fax numbers outside North America are preceded by the international access code ("+") and their country codes (e.g., "+44" for U.K. numbers means that a caller outside the U.K. needs to dial an appropriate international access code followed by "44." Callers within the U.K. would ignore the "+44."). Note also that any leading zero in the city area code is dropped when you dial to another country.

SUPPORT
Cochlear Implants
(See also listing of **Newsletters and Journals** below.)

ACITA
c/o Mr. Yasuo Ogi
6-8-21, Minamikurihara
Zama-City, Kanagawa Prefecture, Japan 228
+81 462 55-0628 (Voice/Fax)

A support group for cochlear implant users and others in Japan. Has over 700 members, 500 with implants. Issues a quarterly newsletter and holds an annual national convention and other small regional events in Japan. ACITA is an acronym for the Association of Cochlear Implant Transmitted Audition. Pronounced "ashita" in Japanese, it also is a Japanese word meaning "tomorrow" or "future hope," and represents the group's optimism about the bright future for cochlear implant users.

Cochlear Implant Club and Advisory Association (CICADA)
c/o Nancy Hoffmann
30 Wongabel Street
Kenmore, Qld, Australia 4069
+61 07 3878-1174 (TTY)
+61 07 3878-9161 (Fax)
ACE.Nancy.Hoffmann@mailbox.uq.edu.au

Australia's national cochlear implant support group. Produces a national newsletter to connect cochlear implant users, families, and others interested in the devices.

Cochlear Implant Club International (CICI)
5335 Wisconsin Avenue N.W., Suite 440
Washington, D.C., U.S.A. 20015 – 2034
(202) 895-2781 (Voice)
(202) 895-2782 (Fax)
http://www.cici.org

This organization provides support, information, and advocacy for those with a cochlear implant or who have an interest in the technology. Members include those with implants, their families, candidates, doctors, audiologists, teachers, scientists, and device manufacturers. Produces a quarterly newsjournal, CONTACT, and mounts a convention every other year. There are chapters of CICI throughout North America, and the office may be able to put you in touch with a local one or help you to form your own. A position paper, "Cochlear Implant Use in Children and Adolescents," is available on request.

Cochlear Implanted Children's Support Group (U.K.):

Southern Region:
Tricia Kemp
4 Ranelagh Avenue
Barnes, London U.K. SW13 0BY
+44 0181 876-8605 (Voice)

Northern Region:
Hilary French
11 Wearside Drive, The Sands
Durham City, U.K. DH1 1LE
+44 0191 386-1112 (Voice)

A United Kingdom group of "parents for parents." The group offers assistance based on first-hand experience of the impact of a cochlear implant on family life and provides information and support for families before, during, and after a child's implant. Provides contacts with other families on a geographical or medical history basis, as well as national and international pen pals for older children.

European Association of Cochlear Implant Users (EURO-CIU)
16, Rue Emile Lavandier
L-1924 Luxembourg
+352 441746 (Voice)
+352 442225 (Fax)

Represents over 1,000 cochlear implant users in fifteen European countries: Norway, Sweden, Germany, Austria, France, Italy, Luxembourg, Belgium, Netherlands, Great Britain, Spain, Portugal, Czechoslovakia, Poland, and Turkey. Members include both cochlear implant associations and individuals from these countries, working to promote consumer information, funding mechanisms, research and development, appropriate training for pedagogical experts, and rehabilitation programs.

National Cochlear Implant Users' Association
692 Bury Road
Bolton BL2 6JD United Kingdom
+44 01204 392196 (Voice)

Formed as a centralized, democratically run national British association to give cochlear implant users a more influential collective voice and to further their interests. The founding president is Lord Jack Ashley of Stoke.

DEAFNESS AND HEARING IMPAIRMENTS

Acoustic Neuroma Association
P.O. Box 12402
Atlanta, GA, U.S.A. 30355
(404) 237-8023 (Voice)
(404) 237-2704 (Fax)
ana.usa@aol.com

Provides support and information for patients who have been diagnosed with or treated for acoustic neuroma or other tumors affecting the cranial nerves. Some members have neurofibromatosis type 2 (NF2) and may be deaf. Some of these people may have received or be candidates for an auditory brainstem implant (ABI), which functions much like a cochlear implant.

Alexander Graham Bell Association for the Deaf
3417 Volta Place N.W.
Washington, D.C., U.S.A. 20007
(202) 337-5220 (Voice/TTY)
agbell2@aol.com
http://www.agbell.org

An association for adults with hearing impairments, parents of people with hearing impairments, and professionals who assist those who are deaf or hard of hearing. The Bell Association has chapters in the United States and Canada, and seven international affiliate organizations. Produces a magazine, *Volta Voices*, six times a year, and a journal, *The Volta Review*, five times a year. Holds conferences that typically have several sessions dealing with cochlear implants. The Bell Association distributes many books and audiovisual materials relating to deafness. Catalog is available on request.

Association of Late-Deafened Adults (ALDA)
10310 Main St., Box 274
Fairfax, VA, U.S.A. 22030
(404) 289-1596 (TTY)
(404) 284-6862 (Fax)

A consumer support organization for adults who became deaf after childhood. Publishes a quarterly newsletter and mounts annual conventions. Chapters throughout the United States.

Canadian Association of the Deaf
2435 Holly Lane, Suite 205
Ottawa, ON, Canada KIV 7P2
(613) 526-4785 (Voice/TTY)
(613) 526-4718 (Fax)

Canadian association of the culturally Deaf. Publishes a bilingual newsletter, *CAD Chat*. Position paper on cochlear implants is available on request.

Canadian Hard of Hearing Association/
L'Association des Malentendants Canadiens
2435 Holly Lane, Suite 205
Ottawa, ON, Canada K1V 7P2
(613) 526-2692 (TTY)
(613) 526-1584 (Voice)
1 800 263-8068 (Voice)
(613) 526-4718 (Fax)
chhanational@cyberus.ca

Canada's only national non-profit consumer organization run by and for hard-of-hearing persons. Chapters and branches across Canada.

Canadian Hearing Society
271 Spadina Road
Toronto, ON, Canada M5R 2V3
(416) 964-9595 (Voice)
(416) 964-0023 (TTY)
(416) 928-2506 (Fax)
http://www.chs.ca
vibeseditor@chs.ca

Provides services such as vocational counselling and sign language training, as well as a store for assistive listening devices for deaf and hard-of-hearing persons throughout the province of Ontario in Canada. Publishes quarterly magazine, *Vibes*. Catalog for assistive devices is available on request.

National Association of the Deaf (NAD)
814 Thayer Avenue
Silver Spring, MD, U.S.A. 20910-4500
(301) 587-1789 (TTY)
(301) 587-1788 (Voice)
(301) 587-1791 (Fax)
NADHQ@juno.com
http://www.nad.org

Since 1880, NAD has existed as an American consumer-based organization representing the deaf – primarily culturally Deaf persons. It has affiliated chapters throughout the United States, holds a biennial national convention, and publishes the monthly periodical, *The NAD Broadcaster*. NAD's position paper on cochlear implants is available on request.

Self Help for Hard of Hearing People, Inc. (SHHH)
7910 Woodmont Avenue, Suite 1200
Bethesda, MD, U.S.A. 20814
(301) 657-2248 (Voice)
(301) 657-2249 (TTY)
(301) 913-9413 (Fax)

http://www.shhh.org
national@shhh.org

The world's largest international consumer organization for hard-of-hearing people, their relatives, and friends. SHHH has chapters throughout the United States (although many members are from outside the United States), organizes regular regional and national conventions at which cochlear implants are typically on the agenda, and publishes a glossy journal, *Hearing Loss*, which frequently covers cochlear implants. The current executive director, Donna L. Sorkin, and the past director and founder, Rocky Stone, both wear cochlear implants.

World Federation of the Deaf
13D Chemin du Levant
F-01210 Ferney-Voltaire, France
+33 4 5040-0107 (Fax)

This organization is made up of members of culturally Deaf associations from many countries. It is in official liaison with the Economic and Social Council of the United Nations UNESCO, ILO, and WHO. The WFD holds congresses every four years. A position paper on cochlear implants is under discussion.

RESEARCH

Boys Town National Research Hospital
555 N. 30th Street
Omaha, NE, U.S.A. 68131
(402) 498-6511 (Voice)
(402) 498-6543 (TTY)
(402) 498-6638 (Fax)
jesteadt@boystown.org
http://www.boystown.org/btnrh

Boys Town conducts research into hereditary hearing loss and maintains a registry of individuals and their families with hereditary hearing loss who are interested in participating in research studies. Other research programs are concerned with the early identification of hearing loss, better hearing-aid fitting, and the consequences of hearing loss for speech and language development. The hospital has developed many materials for the parents of newly identified deaf or hard-of-hearing children, including videotapes on educational options and a sign language training curriculum for parents with young children.

Central Institute for the Deaf (CID) – see entry under **Education and (Re)habilitation**

Cooperative Research Centre for Cochlear Implant, Speech &
   Hearing Research
384-388 Albert Street
East Melbourne, Victoria, Australia 3002
+61 3 9283-7500 (Voice)
+61 3 9283-7518 (Fax)

This center brings together several hearing research groups and biomedical industries to develop and commercialize devices for severe and profound hearing impairments. Its major focus is on cochlear implant research and development. Research for the Nucleus cochlear implant and for the Tickle Talker electrotactile device is conducted here. In addition, the center carries out research to develop speech-processing hearing aids and "combionic" aids (hearing aids that can be used with cochlear implants). Postgraduate research programs and a comprehensive cochlear implant workshop program are offered. The core participants in the center as of 1998 are the Bionic Ear Institute, Australian Hearing Services, Cochlear Limited, and the University of Melbourne.

Deafness Research Foundation
15 West 39th Street
New York, NY, U.S.A. 10018
(212) 768-1181 (Voice/TTY)
(212) 768-1782 (Fax)

The Deafness Research Foundation funds research projects (including projects dealing with cochlear implants) in the United States, Canada, and Puerto Rico. It also sponsors research symposia on the subject of deafness.

Defeating Deafness
330-332 Gray's Inn Road
London, U.K. WC1X 8EE
+44 0171 833-1733 (Voice)
+44 0171 278-0404 (Fax)

Previously known as the Hearing Research Trust, this is the United Kingdom's only medical research charitable organization for deaf and hard-of-hearing people. It provides grants for research into cochlear implants, including a national study (led by scientists at the Institute of Hearing Research in Nottingham) of the effectiveness of cochlear implants in deaf children. The charity was established as a trust in 1985 by Lord Jack and Lady Pauline Ashley of Stoke. Lord Ashley wears a cochlear implant and is a prominent disability advocate in the United Kingdom.

House Ear Institute
2100 West Third Street,
Los Angeles, CA, U.S.A. 90057
(213) 483-4431 (Voice)
(213) 484-2642 (TTY)
(213) 483-8789 (Fax)
Information and Referral Service: 1 800 352-8888 (Voice or TTY), or via numbers listed above
http://www.hei.org

Internationally recognized as a leader in research into ear diseases, balance disorders, and hearing impairments. Research and development of the early single-channel implant took place here. The auditory brainstem implant was developed here, and surgery for auditory brainstem and cochlear implants takes place in the adjacent House Ear Clinic. The institute has a large reference library containing videotapes (including tapings of surgeries), books, and periodicals. Some books, videotapes, and booklets on deafness are available for purchase. The "Lead Line" provides an information and referral service primarily for families with deaf children.

National Institutes of Health
National Institute on Deafness and Other Communication
   Disorders
NIDCD Information Clearinghouse
31 Center Dr. MSC 2320
Bethesda, MD, U.S.A. 20892-2320
"Cochlear Implants Information Package"
(301) 496-7243 (Voice)
http://www.nih.gov/nidcd

National Institutes of Health
U.S. Department of Health and Human Services
Public Health Service
Office of Medical Applications of Research
Building 1, Room 216
Bethesda, MD, U.S.A. 20892
Cochlear Implants in Adults and Children,
Program and Abstracts, and
NIH Consensus Statement
http://consensus.nih.gov

The National Institutes of Health (NIH) is a major funding resource for research into cochlear implants in the United States and elsewhere through its National Institute on Deafness and Other Communication Disorders (NIDCD). For example, the NIH provided financial support to the University of Melbourne in the development of the Nucleus cochlear implant there. The NIH periodically conducts consensus meetings and publishes a consensus statement on cochlear implants as well as the program and abstracts from consensus meetings. The NIDCD Information Clearinghouse distributes the Cochlear Implants Information Package (1996, DC-139), as well as other information on deafness. The *Consensus Statements* and information package are both available on request.

The most recent *Program and Abstracts* resulting from a 1995 consensus meeting is a comprehensive collection of papers on the subject of cochlear implants for adults and children. Papers discuss factors affecting performance, technical and safety considerations, candidacy criteria, and efficacy. Authors include prominent cochlear implant researchers and clinicians working in the United States, Australia, and the United Kingdom. The resulting *Consensus Statement* summarizes these papers.

NIDCD National Temporal Bone, Hearing and Balance Pathology Resource Registry
Massachusetts Eye and Ear Infirmary
243 Charles Street
Boston, MA, U.S.A. 02114-3096
1 800 822-1327 (Voice)
(617) 573-3888 (TTY)
(617) 573-3838 (Fax)
http://www.tbregistry.org

This is a program of the U.S. National Institute on Deafness and Other Communication Disorders (NIDCD). The registry encourages temporal bone (inner ear) donations after death and research using these donations. It works closely with the Deafness Research Foundation and over twenty-five temporal bone research laboratories in the United States.

COCHLEAR IMPLANT SYSTEMS
Advanced Bionics:

Head Office:
Advanced Bionics Corporation
12740 San Fernando Road
Sylmar, CA, U.S.A. 91342
1 800 678-2575 (Voice)
1 800 678-3575 (TTY)
(818) 362-7588 (Outside U.S.A and Canada)
(818) 362-5069 (Fax)
http://www.cochlearimplant.com

Advanced Bionics SARL
13, Avenue Valparc, Bâtiment C
68440 Habsheim/Mulhouse, France
+33 03 89 65 98 00 (Voice)
+33 03 89 65 50 05 (Fax)
info@abionics.fr

Advanced Bionics GmbH
Bahnhofstraße 16
66663 Merzig, Germany
+49 0 6861-5844 (Voice)
+49 0 6861-2741 (Fax)
abionics@t-online.de

Advanced Bionics (U.K.) Ltd.
Grain House, Mill Court
Great Shelford
Cambridge CBZ 5LD U.K.
+44 (0) 1223 847 888 (Voice)
+44 (0) 1223 847 898 (Fax)

Advanced Bionics manufactures the CLARION multichannel implant, which was only the second multichannel cochlear implant device in the United States (after the Cochlear Nucleus) to obtain FDA approval for commercial distribution for adults and children. Approval was granted for adults in 1996, and for children in 1997.

AllHear:

AllHear Inc.
361 Hospital Road
Newport-Lido Medical Building, Suite 327
Newport Beach, CA, U.S.A. 92663
(714) 631-4327 (Voice)
(714) 631-2030 (Fax)
AllHear@cinsight.com
http://www.AllHear.com

Makers of the AllHear single-electrode, all-on-the-head implant system. Owned by Dr. William House, a legendary pioneer in the development of cochlear implants.

Antwerp Bionic Systems:

Head Office:
Antwerp Bionic Systems
Drie Eikenstraat 661
B-2650 Edegem, Belgium
+32 3 825 26 16 (Voice)
+32 3 825 06 30 (Fax)
nick.vanruiten@abs.be
http://www.abs.be/abs

Makers of the LAURA multichannel cochlear implant system. Antwerp Bionic Systems is owned by Philips Hearing Instruments.

Cochlear:

Head Office:
Cochlear Limited
14 Mars Road, P.O. Box 629
Lane Cove, NSW, Australia 2066
+61 2 9428-6555 (Voice)
+61 2 9428-6352 (Fax)

Cochlear Corporation
61 Inverness Drive East, Suite 200
Englewood, CO, U.S.A. 80112
1 800 458-4999
(303) 790-9010 (Voice/TTY)
(303) 792-9025 (Fax)
http://www.cochlear.com

Cochlear AG
Margarethenstrasse 47
CH-4053 Basel, Switzerland
+41 61 205 04 04 (Voice)
+41 61 205 04 05 (Fax)

Cochlear (UK) Ltd.
Mill House, 8 Mill Street
London, U.K. SE1 2BA
+44 171 231-6323 (Voice)
+44 171 231-3371 (Fax)

Nihon Cochlear Co., Ltd.
Kizu Bldg 8th Floor
3-12 Hongo, 3-Chome
Bunkyo-ku, Tokyo 113 Japan
+81 3 3817-0241 (Voice)
+81 3 3817-0245 (Fax)

Cochlear is at this writing the leading cochlear implant manufacturer world-wide measured by numbers of users. It manufactures the Nucleus series of implants and also provides support to users of the Ineraid and the 3M implants, which are no longer produced by their respective manufacturers.

MED-EL:

Headquarters:
MED-EL Medical Electronics
Furstenweg 77a
A6020, Innsbruck, Austria
+43 512 28 88 89 (Voice)
+43 512 29 33 81 (Fax)
office@medel.com
http://www.medel.com

MED-EL Vienna Office
Währinger Strasse 6-8/4/17
A-1090 Wien, Austria
+43 1 31 72 400 (Voice)
+43 1 31 72 4004 (Fax)

MED-EL Deutschland GmbH
Truhenseeweg 2
D-82319 Starnberg, Germany
+49 8151 77 030 (Voice)
+49 8151 77 03 23 (Fax)

MED-EL UK Limited
Bridge Mills, Huddersfield Road
Holmfirth, U.K. HD7 2TW
+44 14 84 68 62 23 (Voice)
+44 14 84 68 60 56 (Fax)

MED-EL Corporation
P.O. Box 14183
Research Triangle Park, NC, U.S.A. 27709
(919) 572-2222 (Voice)
(919) 484-9229 (Fax)

MED-EL Latin America
Sarmiento 212
Buenos Aires, Argentina
+54 1 3452704(05) (Voice)
+54 1 3340166 (Fax)

MED-EL France, SARL
34 Rue de Penthievre
F-75008, Paris, France
+33 1 538 964 45 (Voice)
+33 1 538 964 48 (Fax)

MED-EL Spain
Centro Emprasarial Euronova
C/Ronda de Poniente
16 Bajo L., Spain
+34 1 804-1527 (Voice)
+34 1 804-4348 (Fax)

Makers of the Combi-40 and Combi 40+ multichannel implants, and the Comfort Implant System single-channel implant. MED-EL's devices are the second most common cochlear implant devices used in Europe, after the Cochlear Nucleus.

MXM:

Head Office:
MXM Medical Technologies
2720 Chemin Saint-Bernard
F-06224 Vallauris Cedex, France
+33 4 93 95 18 18 (Voice)
+33 4 93 95 38 01 (Fax)
digisonic@mxmlab.com
http:// www.mxmlab.com

MXM Medizinische Implantate GmbH
Mainzer Straße 116
D-66121 Saarbrucken, Germany
+49 681 99 63 0 (Voice)
+49 681 99 63 111 (Fax)

Makers of the Digisonic multichannel cochlear implant and auditory brainstem implant. The Digisonic is available in Europe, Saudi Arabia, and the Middle East.

EDUCATION AND (RE)HABILITATION

American Speech-Language-Hearing Association (ASHA)
10801 Rockville Pike
Rockville, MD, U.S.A. 20852
(301) 897-5700 (Voice/TTY)
1 800 638-8255 (Voice TTY 8:30 a.m. - 5:00 p.m. Eastern Time)
(301) 571-0457 (Fax)
irc@asha.org
http://www.asha.org

ASHA is the professional, scientific, and credentialing association for more than 90,000 audiologists, speech-language pathologists, and speech, language, and hearing scientists. The association publishes materials for professionals, including five journals, and makes a series of brochures, fact sheets, and information packets (including a cochlear implant information package) available to the general public at no cost. It also provides consumers with referrals to professionals and programs.

Auditory-Verbal International (AVI)
2121 Eisenhower Avenue, Suite 402
Alexandria, VA, U.S.A. 22314
(703) 739-1049 (Voice)
(703) 739-0874 (TTY)
(703) 739-0395 (Fax)

AVI is dedicated to ensuring that all children with hearing impairments who have the potential to develop speech and language through hearing have the opportunity to do so. It publishes a professional code of ethics for auditory-verbal therapists, certifies qualified therapists, and organizes regular conferences. Publishes a quarterly newsletter, *The Auricle,* and a bimonthly parent newsletter, *Backtalk!,* with a pull-out children's section.

Boys Town National Research Hospital: see entry above under **Research**.

Central Institute for the Deaf (CID)
818 South Euclid Avenue
St. Louis, MO, U.S.A. 63110-1594
(314) 977-0000 (Voice/TTY)
(314) 977-0025 (Fax)
bf@cidmac.wustl.edu
http://cidmac.wustl.edu/

The CID is a private, non-profit institute that conducts research into the normal aspects as well as the disorders of hearing, language, and speech, and has a school for children who have hearing impairments. It has speech, language, and hearing clinics; it offers professional education programs in audiology, education of persons with hearing impairments, and communication sciences. The institute conducts studies of students with cochlear implants attending the school, as well as children with cochlear implants across the United States and Canada in a variety of educational settings. The CID distributes professional and consumer brochures and educational materials, as well as *News Notes*, a professional and consumer newsletter.

Cochlear Implant Training Institute (CITI)
League for the Hard of Hearing
71 West 23rd Street
New York, NY, U.S.A. 10010-4162
(212) 741-6073 (Voice)
(212) 255-1932 (TTY)
(212) 255-4413 (Fax)
http://www.lhh.org

CITI is a national resource center on rehabilitation for children with cochlear implants. It will provide assistance on request to parents of children who have received or are considering a cochlear implant, and to professionals working with these children. It offers help with the assessment of language, speaking and listening skills, planning for customized rehabilitation programs for children, and in-service training for educational and support staff.

Cochlear Implants International
246a Willoughby Rd.
Naremburn, NSW, Australia 2065
+61 612 9439-7566 (Voice)
+61 612 9439-7415 (Fax)
gibsonwp@onaustralia.com.au

Supports hearing-impaired children and adults in the Asian region, from bases in Australia and Singapore. Conducts assessments for cochlear implant surgery and provides surgery and post-operative services. Clients in Hong Kong, Sri Lanka, Philippines, Malaysia, Singapore, Indonesia, Bangladesh, and Dubai.

Cued Speech:

National Cued Speech Association

Nazareth College of Rochester

4245 East Avenue,

Rochester, NY, U.S.A. 14618

(716) 389-2776 (Voice)

(716) 586-2452 (Fax)

NCSA@naz.edu

Cued Speech Discovery

National Cued Speech Association Information Service/Bookstore

23970 Hermitage Road

Cleveland, OH, U.S.A. 44122-4008

1 800 459-3529 (Voice/TTY)

(216) 292-6213 (Voice/TTY)

cuedspdisc@aol.com

Cued speech, which uses different hand shapes in different locations near the mouth to distinguish between sounds that look alike, can be an effective supplement to lipreading, while improving lipreading skills. The rise of Deaf pride and ASL has to some extent made it less popular in North America, and it is more commonly used in Europe. In France, it is often used with children before they get a cochlear implant, and for a period of time thereafter. Information and referrals can be obtained by contacting Cued Speech Discovery.

The Ear Foundation

c/o Nottingham Pediatric Cochlear Implant Programme

113 The Ropewalk

Nottingham, U.K. NG1 6HA

+44 0115 948-5549 (Voice)

+44 0115 948-5560 (Fax)

Provides a family support and rehabilitation center in Nottingham. Offers information for teachers and other professionals working in the field and acts as a national and international resource center.

Also supports the work of the Cochlear Implanted Children's Support Group in the United Kingdom. (See above, under **Support**.) The Nottingham Pediatric Cochlear Implant Programme published a progress report in 1997 on implant efficacy (available on request) that it says is based on the largest body of data on young implanted children from any single institution in the world.

Gallaudet University
National Information Center on Deafness
800 Florida Avenue N.E.
Washington, D.C., U.S.A. 20002-3695
(202) 651-5052 (TTY)
(202) 651-5051 (Voice)
(202) 651-5054 (Fax)
nicd@gallux.gallaudet.edu
http://www.gallaudet.edu/~nicd

Gallaudet is the world's only four-year liberal arts university for students who are deaf or hard of hearing. Its National Information Center on Deafness provides extensive consumer information on deafness (and some material on cochlear implants) on request.

HEAR NOW
9745 East Hamden Avenue, Suite 300
Denver, CO, U.S.A. 80231-4923
(303) 695-7797 or 1 800 648-HEAR (Voice/TTY)

HEAR NOW is a U.S. charitable organization that provides hearing aids and cochlear implants and related services for hearing-impaired adults and children who need them but are unable to finance them on their own.

Hearing Rehabilitation Foundation
35 Medford Street,
Somerville, MA, U.S.A. 02143
(617) 628-4537 (Voice)
(617) 258-7003 (Fax)
plant@cbgrle.mit.edu

This organization produces extensive rehabilitative materials for deaf persons and their therapists. The founder, Geoff Plant, also offers rehabilitative services to individuals. Most of the material was developed for hearing-impaired adults in general and is applicable to those with a cochlear implant.

Helen Keller National Center for Deaf-Blind Youths and Adults
111 Middle Neck Road
Sands Point, NY, U.S.A. 11055
(516) 944-8900 (Voice)
(516) 944-8637 (TTY)
(516) 944-7302 (Fax)
abigailp@aol.com

Provides comprehensive evaluation and training with an emphasis on job preparation and independent living for people who are both deaf and blind. Offers information and referral, advocacy, technical assistance, and training to professionals, consumers, and families.

John Tracy Clinic
806 West Adams Boulevard
Los Angeles, CA, U.S.A. 90007
1 800 522-4582 (Voice/TTY)
(213) 748-5481 (Voice)
(213) 747-2924 (TTY)

This clinic provides a correspondence course on rehabilitation for parents and educators of hearing-impaired children, from birth to five years of age.

The Listening Center at Johns Hopkins
P.O. Box 41402
Baltimore, MD, U.S.A. 21203-6402
(410) 955-9397 (Voice/TTY)
(410) 614-9167 (Fax)

Provides on-site rehabilitation services for children with cochlear implants through weekly therapy sessions and computer-based training exercises designed to speed auditory processing and promote language acquisition. The center offers parent training in workshops and support groups; educational support in the child's school; and professional training through seminars and a videotape series. Accepts selected adult implant users into the program.

National Adult Cochlear Implant Rehabilitation Center (NACIRC)
League for the Hard of Hearing
71 West 23rd Street
New York, NY, U.S.A. 10010-4162
(212) 741-7697 (Voice)
(212) 255-1932 (TTY)
(212) 255-4413 (Fax)
http://www.lhh.org

The NACIRC provides services to adults to maximize the communication benefits they receive from a cochlear implant. After evaluation, an individual program may be devised that includes auditory training, speechreading, English as a Second Language training, speech and voice therapy, self-advocacy and communication strategies. The league has a hearing museum on hearing impairment open to group tours on appointment and has a catalog (available on request) listing publications, videotapes, and audiotapes.

Network of Educators of Children with Cochlear Implants (NECCI)
Cochlear Implant Center
Lenox Hill Hospital
186 East 76th Street
New York, NY, U.S.A. 10021
(212) 434-2000 (Voice)
PMChute@aol.com

NECCI is an organization for professionals involved in the education of children with cochlear implants. Publishes a newsletter, *NECCI News*, and curriculum materials to train other professionals regarding cochlear implants.

New Zealand Cochlear Implant Program
98 Remuera Road
Auckland, New Zealand 5
+64 09 520-4009 (Voice)
+64 09 522-1622 (Fax)
cdevlin@ahsl.co.nz

The base for the national cochlear implant program in New Zealand. See also *Cochlear Implant Newsletter* under **Newsletters and Journals**.

Resource Point
61 Inverness Drive East, Suite 200
Englewood, CO, U.S.A. 80112
1 800 688-8788 (Voice/TTY: U.S. and Canada)
(303) 790-9010 (Voice/TTY: all other countries)
(303) 792-9025 (Fax)

This is the publication division of Cochlear Corporation, makers of the Nucleus cochlear implant system. It produces and markets rehabilitation materials, including speech production skills testing materials, classroom curricula, and computer software packages for use with hearing-impaired children, as well as adults.

VOICE for Hearing Impaired Children
124 Eglinton Ave. West, Suite 420
Toronto, ON, Canada, M4R 2G8
(416) 487-7719 (Voice/TTY)
(416) 487-7423 (Fax)
voice@web.net
http://www.web.net/~voice

An advocacy and support group for families with hearing-impaired children. Offers auditory-verbal therapy to children and trains therapists. Chapters throughout the Canadian province of Ontario, and in a few other Canadian provinces as well.

NEWSLETTERS AND JOURNALS

(Note that many of the organizations listed above produce newsletters and journals for members. See also the entry for **MEDLINE** under the **Internet** listings.)

Cochlear Implant Newsletter
c/o Lynsey Farra
2 Liestrella Road
Christchurch, New Zealand 2
+64 3 338-9988 (Voice/Fax)

A newsletter for cochlear implant users, families, and others in New Zealand.

Hearing Health
P.O. Drawer V
Ingleside, TX, U.S.A. 78362-0500
(512) 776-7240 (Voice/TTY)
(512) 776-3278 (Fax)

A consumer magazine that calls itself "The Voice on Hearing Issues." The current editor, Paula Bonillas, is an enthusiastic user of a cochlear implant. You may write to request a free sample issue.

HiP Magazine
1563 Solano Avenue, #137
Berkeley, CA, U.S.A. 94707
(510) 527-8993 (Voice)
(510) 527-9088 (Fax)

A magazine for kids with a hearing loss, aged eight through four-teen. Full of pizzaz, with interesting articles, not all of which are related to deafness. A recent issue had articles on the Internet, snakes, the National Theater of the Deaf, and Linda Bove. Bound to encourage positive feelings about hearing impairment in kids. Published six times a year and comes with a companion teaching guide called *HiP TiPs*.

Life After Deafness
6773 Starboard Way
Sacramento, CA, U.S.A. 95831-2413

A bimonthly magazine published by two late-deafened adults (one of whom, Gayle McCullough, wears a cochlear implant), on the subject of – as the title indicates – living with deafness.

The NF2 Review
c/o The House Ear Institute
2100 West Third Street, 2nd Floor
Los Angeles, CA, U.S.A. 90057
(213) 483-4431 (Voice)
(213) 484-2642 (TTY)
(213) 413-0950 (Fax)
bgxg89a@prodigy.com

A newsletter providing current information about research and treatment of neurofibromatosis type 2, as well as personal experi-ence articles. Frequent items on the subject of auditory brainstem implants (ABIs).

Pacific Northwest Cochlear Implant Newsletter
26820 Arden Court
Kent, WA, U.S.A. 98032
(253) 854-0171 (Voice/TTY)
Gordon_Nystedt@msn.com

Produced four times a year by a cochlear implant user, and distributed to over 450 subscribers. Although there is no subscription fee, a donation to help cover the cost of printing and mailing is appreciated. The newsletter is aimed at all implantees (regardless of where they live), as well as those interested in learning more about cochlear implants. Carries many personal testimonials.

Schnecke (Leben mit dem Cochlear Implant)
Deutsche Cochlear Implant Gesellschaft e. V.
Siegfried-Ott-Str. 4
D-89257 Illertissen, Germany
http://ourworld.compuserve.com/homepages/mhh_hno

A glossy magazine in German for cochlear implant users, families, teachers, professionals, and others with an interest in cochlear implants in Germany and other states in Europe where German is spoken. It is published by the Deutsche Cochlear Implant Gesellschaft e.V. (German cochlear implant society). The current editors, Hanna Hermann and Wolfard Grascha, are themselves cochlear implant users.

Silent News
133 Gaither Dr., Suite E
Mt. Laurel, NJ, U.S.A. 08054-1710

A monthly newspaper that describes itself as the "world's most popular newspaper of deaf and hard-of-hearing people."

TUNE-INternational
c/o Sue Archbold
Nottingham Pediatric Cochlear Implant Centre
113 The Ropewalk
Nottingham, U.K. NG1 6HA

This is an international newsletter published in the United Kingdom for children with cochlear implants and their families. It is distributed by Cochlear U.K. Ltd.

AUDIO-VISUAL RESOURCES

(Note that some cochlear implant device manufacturers produce and distribute videotapes about adults and children with cochlear implants. See individual listings under **Cochlear Implant Systems**.)

Learning to Hear Again
University of Utah
Clough Shelton M.D.
Division of Otolaryngology - HNS
50 N. Medical Drive, 3C120
Salt Lake City, UT, U.S.A. 84132
(801) 585-5450 (Voice)
(801) 585-5744 (Fax)

A series of practice videotapes designed for use by adventitiously deafened adult cochlear implant recipients. All narrated portions of the tapes are open-captioned.

Sound Hearing
by S. Harold Collins
Distributed by:
Harris Communications
15 159 Technology Drive
Eden Prairie, MN, U.S.A. 55344
1 800 825-0564 (Voice)
1 800 551-4118 (TTY)

(612) 906-1099 (Fax)
http://www.harriscomm.com
mail@harriscomm.com.

This audiotape and accompanying booklet explain (and show) what it's like to be hearing impaired. A hearing person listening to the tape will hear music and speech imperfectly – much like hearing-impaired people do.

Summer's Song
c/o Linda Bittner Crider
1030 S.W. 11th Terrace
Gainesville, FL, U.S.A. 32601
Summer (aged 13): sucrider@aol.com
Linda: LBCrider@aol.com

This videotape presents a mother's story about her hearing-impaired daughter, who was deafened by meningitis at the age of three, and implanted at the age of six.

INTERNET
MEDLINE AND THE "INTERNET GRATEFUL MED"
MEDLINE is an excellent source of information on cochlear implants. It is the U.S. National Library of Medicine's premier bibliographic database covering the fields of medicine, nursing, dentistry, veterinary medicine, the health care system, and the preclinical sciences. The MEDLINE database contains bibliographic citations and author abstracts from over 3,800 current biomedical journals published in the United States and seventy foreign countries, from 1966 to the present.

I access this database through the University of Toronto, both online via the Internet, and at the university library itself. Most university libraries provide access to MEDLINE. Access to the online database is also available free to the public through the "Internet Grateful Med," a product of the U.S. National Library of Medicine. The program offers assisted searching in MEDLINE and other databases created by the National Library of Medicine. To access this excellent search tool and database, and its companion, PUBMED, point your World Wide Web browser at:

http://www.nlm.nih.gov/databases/freemedl.html

or go directly to:

http://igm.nlm.nih.gov/

DISCUSSION GROUPS, FORUMS

Sociologist Lee Sproull of Boston University, who has been studying the social value of online support groups, says they provide us with access to "scarce social attention." Several discussion groups on the Internet and commercial online services deal with deafness. Many include exchanges about cochlear implants, and participants are typically generous in sharing information about their experiences. These groups allow deaf people to extend their community (which may contain few deaf people, and even fewer cochlear implant users) to encompass the whole online world. Here are a few groups:

AOL CICI Chat Room:
A chat room on the commercial information service, America Online (AOL), for members and friends of Cochlear Implant Club International (CICI). From the Welcome screen, select *People Connection*. You will enter a general "lobby," and from there you can select *Private Room*. Once there, type in "CICI" and hit enter to go to the CICI Chat Room.

AOL PC Pals Teen Network:
A message board on the Deaf and Hard of Hearing Forum of America Online (AOL). Information is available on the World Wide Web (WWW) at:
http://www.agbell.org/programs/pcpals.html

Beyond-Hearing:
A very warm and supportive group dealing with hearing impairment: a real online community. The moderator firmly keeps the

group and the discussion in-line. Send a message to
majordomo@acpub.duke.edu
with a blank subject line, and the following text in the body of the
message (without the quotes):
"subscribe beyond-hearing"

CI Forum:
Devoted to issues related to cochlear implants. Send a message to
listserv@yorku.ca
with a blank subject line, and the following text in the body of the
message (without the quotes, and using your real name):
"subscribe ci yourfirstname yourlastname"

CompuServe Deaf/Hard of Hearing Section:
A message board on the Disabilities Forum of the commercial infor-
mation service, CompuServe. Many participants have cochlear
implants or are parents of children with cochlear implants. Within
CompuServe, "join" the Disabilities Forum, then proceed to the
Deaf/Hard of Hearing Section to participate.

The NF2 Crew:
A private online group for people with neurofibromatosis type 2
(NF2), and their families. Functions as a place of support and cam-
eraderie, and a place to share information. To join or find out more
about the group, send a message to Jordan Anne Harlow at
jdharlow@aol.com
or Jennette Braaten at
jennette@cdsnet.net.

SayWhatClub Forum:
A chatty discussion group; a friend calls it "a set of training wheels
for hearing loss." Contact
info@saywhatclub.com
for details.

WORLD WIDE WEB

You can obtain a great deal of information here by simply doing a search using one of the WWW search engines (such as that found at http://altavista.digital.com/) using the search term "cochlear implant" (include the quote marks to indicate that you want matches of both words "cochlear" and "implant" together). A Net search will turn up many more, but a few good WWW sites with comprehensive cochlear implant-related information are:

http://weber.u.washington.edu/~otoweb/cochlear_implants.html
http://www.ears.com
http://www.tsi.it/contrib/audies/impianti.html

The following WWW sites are excellent ones for parents of newly diagnosed deaf and hard-of-hearing children:

http://www.gohear.org
http://members.tripod.com/~listenup/

Search the Internet for current discussion groups related to deafness and/or cochlear implants other than the ones listed above at the following WWW site:

http:www.liszt.com

There are over 70,000 discussion groups (on all topics) from which to choose.

Or search for an Internet newsgroup by topic or name at the following WWW site:

http://tile.net/news/bitl112.html

There are over 15,000 newsgroups available covering a very wide range of topics.

RECOMMENDED READING

This is a highly selective and personal listing of books on the subject of deafness and cochlear implants. See also the Endnotes and the Resources listing for references to other books, as well as articles, newsletters, and journals.

Ackehurst, Shirley. *Broken Silence.* Sydney: Collins, 1989.
Now out of print, this book is a memoir by an Australian woman, recounting her experiences with her cochlear implant.

Allum, Dianne J., ed. *Cochlear Implant Rehabilitation in Children and Adults.* San Diego: Singular Publishing, 1996.
International in scope, with reports from clinics in Russia, France, Germany, Australia, Spain, the United Kingdom and other countries. A recurring theme is that rehabilitation programs in some form do help cochlear implant recipients, both adults and children.

Ashley, Lord Jack. *Journey into Silence.* London: Bodley Head, 1973.
An autobiography by the British parliamentarian who became deaf while serving as a member of parliament. He later obtained a cochlear implant and became a prominent activist for the rights of those with disabilities.

Clark, Graeme M.; Cowan, Robert S.C.; and Dowell, Richard C., eds. *Cochlear Implantation for Infants and Children: Advances.* San Diego: Singular Publishing, 1997.
The cover photo of four-year-old Tommy is almost worth the price of the book. Tommy received a cochlear implant at the age of twenty-two months, and is now fluent in both English and Croatian. According to the description, Tommy "can communicate easily without the need to lipread and his voice is of normal quality." This 1997 book contains a comprehensive collection of

articles by the Melbourne, Australia team, with an emphasis on the Nucleus 22 and Nucleus 24 devices. Parents considering a cochlear implant for their child will find much of interest in this book, including case studies. The chapter "Ethical Issues" is a thorough treatment of the ethics of cochlear implantation.

Clark, Graeme M.; Tong, Yit C.; and Patrick, James F., eds. *Cochlear Prostheses*. Edinburgh: Churchill Livingstone, 1990.
A well-illustrated, comprehensive (and technical) treatment of the subject, drawing on work carried out at the University of Melbourne and Cochlear Limited in Australia. Excellent material on the development of the Melbourne prototype prosthesis, which was later commercially developed as the Nucleus by Cochlear. The paper on the surgery of cochlear implantation and its accompanying illustrations are especially interesting.

Cohen, Leah Hager. *Train Go Sorry: Inside a Deaf World*. Boston: Houghton Mifflin, 1994.
A story of the yearning of a hearing woman to be deaf. Cohen's father was the superintendent of the Lexington School for the Deaf in New York City.

Cooper, Huw, ed. *Cochlear Implants: A Practical Guide*. San Diego: Singular Publishing, 1991.
This is one of my favorite, comprehensive treatments of the subject. Not aimed at the lay reader, but highly readable nonetheless. Be forewarned, however, that some of the discussions of the devices and performance levels may be out of date.

Davis, Hallowell, and Silverman, S. Richard. *Hearing and Deafness*. 4th ed. New York: Holt, Rinehart and Winston, 1978.
A classic textbook on the subject, for a good reason. It is comprehensive and well-written.

Epstein, June. *The Story of the Bionic Ear*. Melbourne: Hyland House, 1989.
> The story of the development and use of the first multichannel implant in Australia. Includes personal experience stories of implant users.

Estabrooks, Warren, ed. *Auditory-Verbal Therapy for Parents and Professionals*. Washington, D.C.: Alexander Graham Bell Association for the Deaf, 1994.
> A highly readable description of this therapy for hearing-impaired children. The personal stories written by parents of children with cochlear implants are wonderful.

Gannon, Jack R. *Deaf Heritage: A Narrative History of Deaf America*. Silver Spring, Maryland: National Association of the Deaf, 1981.
> Reading through this encyclopedia, with its lists of Deaf firsts (first Deaf pilot, first Deaf Baptist minister), its list of high-achieving Deaf people (Deaf people with earned doctorate degrees, Deaf people in the arts), and famous children of Deaf parents, it is possible to get a sense of a real community of the Deaf who sign.

Glennie, Evelyn. *Good Vibrations*. Long Preston: Magna Print, 1991.
> An autobiography by the accomplished Scottish deaf percussionist.

Golan, Lew. *Reading Between the Lips: A Totally Deaf Man Makes It in the Mainstream*. Chicago: Bonus Books, 1995.
> The title says it all. An autobiography that takes a humorous look at growing up oral deaf.

Grant, Brian, ed. *The Quiet Ear: Deafness in Literature*. London: Andre Deutsch, 1987.

An interesting compilation of literary excerpts on the subject of deafness. Includes a poignant excerpt by Turgenev about the deaf serf, Gerasim; Beethoven's description of his despair at being deaf; David Wright's eloquent writing on the experience of deafness.

Heppner, Cheryl M. *Seeds of Disquiet: One Deaf Woman's Experience*. Washington, D.C.: Gallaudet University Press, 1992.

A beautifully and honestly written autobiography by a disability activist who was deafened by meningitis at the age of six.

Kisor, Henry. *What's That Pig Outdoors? A Memoir of Deafness*. New York: Penguin, 1990.

A funny and moving account of growing up deaf by the book review editor of the *Chicago Sun-Times*.

Lane, Harlan. *The Mask of Benevolence: Disabling the Deaf Community*. New York: Alfred A. Knopf, 1992.

Lane is the leading spokesperson in the English language for the Deaf culture, and is opposed to cochlear implants for children. His books on deafness, including this one, are crammed with polemic, anger, and history. Lane has been known to lament that members of the Deaf culture (Lane is hearing) don't read his books.

Lang, Harry G. *Silence of the Spheres*. Westport, Connecticut: Bergin & Garvey, 1994.

A history of science, from a special angle: one that focuses on scientists who are or were deaf. Lang uses Jerome Schein's definition of the deaf as those who "cannot carry on a conversation with their eyes closed" to include both deaf and Deaf in his history. An eloquently penned, fascinating account.

Lang, Harry G., and Meath-Lang, Bonnie. *Deaf Persons in the Arts and Sciences: A Biographical Dictionary*. Westport, Conn.: Greenwood Press, 1995.
>   Profiles of Beethoven, Edison, Smetana, Goya, Ruth Benedict, Henry Kisor, Frances Woods, Bernard Bragg, and many more deaf people who have made their mark in the arts and sciences.

Lovley, Shawn. *Now What? Life After Deaf*. Published by the author, 1996 (2812 Nomad Court West, Bowie, MD 20716, U.S.A.).
>   Lovley suddenly lost all his hearing in 1990, and this book, like that of Bena Shuster's, tries to make the way easier for others in a similar (all-too-often devastating) situation.

Luterman, David M. with Ross, Mark. *When Your Child Is Deaf: A Guide for Parents*. Parkton, Maryland: York Press, 1991.
>   A helpful guide for parents that delves into the issue of coping skills, of guilt, of "loving the child's deafness," and many more complex issues. Includes practical information on hearing tests, hearing aids, and assistive listening devices.

MacKinnon, Christy. *Silent Observer*. Fredericton, N.B.: Goose Lane, 1995.
>   A charming children's book, with lovely illustrations, and an appealing true story of a woman born in 1889 in Nova Scotia, who became deaf at the age of two from a bout of whooping cough. In spite of the sadness, there is also much that is positive in this story. For children of all ages.

Merker, Hannah. *Listening*. New York: Harper Collins, 1994.
>   A dreamy, introspective, often poetic look at living with deafness.

Nevins, Mary Ellen, and Chute, Patricia M. *Children with Cochlear Implants in Educational Settings*. San Diego: Singular Publishing Group, 1996.

Practical advice for professionals working with children, as well
as for parents, in how to develop programs to maximize the
potential of a cochlear implant. Includes useful glossaries and
equipment trouble-shooting guides.

Orlans, Harold, ed. *Adjustment to Adult Hearing Loss.* San Diego:
College-Hill Press, 1985.
An excellent collection of articles on the psychological and soci-
ological aspects of deafness that occurs in adulthood.

Owens, Elmer, and Kessler, Dorcas K., eds. *Cochlear Implants in Young
Deaf Children.* Boston: College-Hill Press, 1989.
An early and thought-provoking coverage of the issues involved
in implanting children. Although much more is now known
about how well children can actually do with implants, the issues
discussed remain pertinent.

Padden, Carol, and Humphries, Tom. *Deaf in America: Voices from a
Culture.* Cambridge: Harvard University Press, 1988.
An enjoyable look at Deaf culture and American Sign Language,
with stories, anecdotes, discussions of Deaf theater, and tran-
scriptions of signed poetry.

Parasnis, Ila, ed. *Cultural and Language Diversity and the Deaf
Experience.* Cambridge: Cambridge University Press, 1996.
A fine collection of essays, some providing an intimate view of
the Deaf culture.

Peterson, Kevin R. *Our Spark of Hope.* Lindborg, Kansas: Carlsons',
1989.
A father's story about his child's experience in becoming deaf
from meningitis, and then becoming one of the first children in
the world to receive a multichannel implant in 1987.

Rees, Jessica. *Sing a Song of Silence: A Deaf Girl's Odyssey*. London: Kensal Press, 1986.

The first autobiography of a deaf person that I really identified with. Poignant and beautifully written. Rees received an early five-electrode implant in England in 1984, after she completed this book.

Sacks, Oliver. *Seeing Voices: A Journey into the World of the Deaf*. Berkeley: University of California Press, 1989.

Sacks's infectious enthusiasm for the subject spills over into copious footnotes. A highly sympathetic yet at the same time distanced look at Deaf culture.

Salvi, Richard J.; Henderson, Donald; Fiorino, Franco; and Colletti, Vittorio, eds. *Auditory System Plasticity and Regeneration*. New York: Thieme, 1996.

A collection of papers discussing the status of research into auditory system plasticity. Includes papers on ear hair cell regeneration, the effects of deafness and electrical stimulation on the auditory system, and a discussion of cochlear implant performance over time as an indicator of auditory system plasticity in humans. While this is not meant as a book for the lay reader, and portions are written in highly technical language, it can be rewarding to a lay reader with a serious interest in the subject.

Schindler, Robert A., and Merzenich, Michael A., eds. *Cochlear Implants*. New York: Raven Press, 1985.

Based on the Proceedings of the Tenth Anniversary Conference on Cochlear Implants, June 22 to 24, 1983, at the University of California, San Francisco. The historical papers by Drs. House, Simmons, and Michelson are especially interesting. This conference took place when the field was just taking off.

Shuster, Bena. *Life after Deafness: A Resource Book for Late-Deafened Adults.* Ottawa: Canadian Hard of Hearing Association, 1995.

> Shuster became deaf overnight as the result of a viral infection. She has written this resource book to help ensure that others in a similar position will not need to endure the terrible confusion and lack of information she was faced with then.

Sidransky, Ruth. *In Silence: Growing up Hearing in a Deaf World.* New York: Ballantine, 1990.

> The anger of Sidransky's parents at their deafness, their rage, is often palpable in this tenderly written book by their hearing daughter. Sidransky was initially placed in a class for retarded children, because her Deaf speech was so poor. As wonderful a writer as she is, she still considers her first language, sign language, to be the language in which she can be most eloquent.

Storr, Anthony. *Music and the Mind.* New York: MacMillan, 1992.

> A popular account by a British psychiatrist of the effect of music on our minds (and bodies). His descriptions of the effect of sound deprivation on those who are deaf have the ring of truth to them.

Thomsett, Kay, and Nickerson, Eve. *Missing Words: The Family Handbook on Adult Hearing Loss.* Washington, D.C.: Gallaudet University Press, 1993.

> An intriguing book written by a mother deafened in adulthood, and her hearing daughter. Has some good communication tips for those newly deafened.

Tucker, Bonnie Poitras. *The Feel of Silence.* Philadelphia: Temple University Press, 1995.

> An eloquent memoir of a deaf woman who has succeeded in a hearing world. Tucker's account of her marriage and divorce (her husband grew tired of her deafness) is chilling.

Tye-Murray, Nancy. *Cochlear Implants & Children: A Handbook for Parents, Teachers & Speech & Hearing Professionals.* Washington, D.C.: Alexander Graham Bell Association, 1993.

> A collection of articles covering a wide variety of topics related to cochlear implants, with a basic theme of helping the child to get the best use out of his or her implant system.

Tyler, Richard S., ed. *Cochlear Implants: Audiological Foundations.* San Diego: Singular Publishing, 1993.

> A comprehensive treatment of the subject by leading experts in the field. While it is not written for the lay person, interested lay readers may still find it understandable and helpful.

Walker, Lou Ann. *A Loss for Words: The Story of Deafness in a Family.* New York: Harper, 1986.

> A sensitive account of what it is like to grow up hearing with deaf parents. It's hard not to like and empathize with this author. Walker's story made me take a second look at my own sister's life. Growing up with a deaf father and deaf sister undoubtedly had a huge effect on her.

Wright, David. *Deafness.* New York: Stein and Day, 1975.

> A beautifully written autobiography by a British poet who was deafened by scarlet fever at the age of seven. Includes a good survey of the history of the education of the deaf.

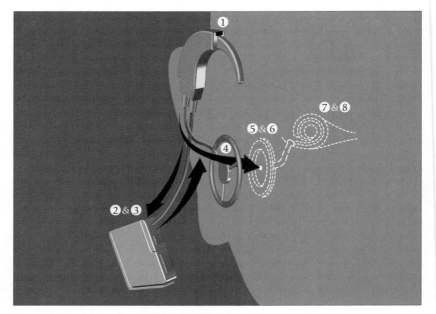

Figure 1: Author's Cochlear Implant System*

1. Sound is received by microphone.
2. Sound is sent from microphone to speech processor.
3. Speech processor translates sound into electrical codes.
4. Codes are sent back to the transmitter.
5. Transmitter sends codes across skin to receiver/stimulator.
6. Receiver/stimulator converts codes to electrical signals.
7. Electrical signals are sent to electrode array within cochlea to stimulate neurons.
8. Neurons send messages along auditory nerve to the central auditory system in the brain where they are interpreted as sound.

---

*This is a description of the author's implant system. While the basic principles of operation are similar for all multichannel devices commercially available in 1998, the components may vary in size and appearance, and certain components (e.g., the microphone and transmitter) may be combined. A behind-the-ear processor currently in clinical trials in several countries shrinks the size of the processor, moves it to ear level, and combines it with the microphone.

INDEX

Sidenotes and endnotes are indicated by a page ref. with an "n" preceding the note number.